Healing the
Anxiety Diseases

Healing the Anxiety Diseases

Thomas L. Leaman, M.D.

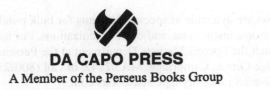

DA CAPO PRESS
A Member of the Perseus Books Group

Library of Congress Cataloging-in-Publication Data is available

ISBN 0-7382-0873-6

Da Capo Press is a Member of the Perseus Books Group.

Find us on the World Wide Web at http://www.dacapopress.com

Da Capo Press books are available at special discounts for bulk purchases in the U.S. by corporations, institutions, and other organizations. For more information, please contact the Special Markets Department at the Perseus Books Group, 11 Cambridge Center, Cambridge, MA 02142, or call (800)255-1514 or (617)252-5298, or e-mail j.mccrary@perseusbooks.com.

First paperback printing, December 2002

10 9 8 7 6 5 4

To my beloved Jeanne

Acknowledgments

The inspiration for this book came from my patients, especially Ruth, Robert, Paul, and Henrietta, and to them I will always owe a debt of gratitude for my education in anxiety diseases. For her typing, and her patience with the many retypings, I thank my friend and secretary, Carol Jackson. For the lessons in grammar, for the creative ideas, and for the poking and prodding, I thank my literary consultant and agent, my daughter, Rebecca Pratt. And I especially thank my wife, Jeanne, who has supported and encouraged me in this and everything I've done.

                                        Thomas L. Leaman, M.D.

Hershey, Pennsylvania

Contents

The guilty flee when no man pursueth.
Proverbs

Chapter 1

Anxiety Disease
There Is Good News

Have you ever experienced repeated drenching sweats, or been plagued by persistent fatigue for no apparent reason? Stomach cramps? Headaches? Rapid heartbeat? Chest pain? Shortness of breath? Endless sleepless nights? Have you ever felt like a hostage in your own home? Are you afraid to leave the safety of those familiar walls? Have you ever said, "It's just my nerves. I'll be fine as soon as things settle down and I get myself together. It's probably my own fault. I should have taken that vacation when I had the chance."

If none of these descriptions apply directly to you, then certainly one out of every dozen or so people that you know, and possibly someone you care about very deeply, has suffered from a handful of these symptoms of misery.

A 1982 study by the prestigious National Institute of Mental Health (NIMH) showed that more than 9.5% of the American public suffered from anxiety disease within the six months prior to the survey. This means that almost one out of every ten people experienced these painful symptoms during that period. Over an individual's lifetime, the percentages will, of course, be far higher.

This same study revealed another astonishing fact: only twenty-three percent of those 13 million people have sought treatment. The remaining three-fourths—that's 9,750,000 people—suffer the misery of anxiety disease and its consequences of disrupted relationships and unhappiness without seeking help of any kind.

Why? These results came as such a surprise that the study wasn't even designed to answer this question. The most probable explanation, I believe, lies in the nature of the anxiety diseases themselves and in how people perceive them. There are many widespread beliefs about anxiety disease and most of them are dead wrong. These mistaken assumptions keep people from looking for the help they so desperately need.

One deeply ingrained belief is that all anxiety problems are caused by stress or, at least, are a reaction to stress. It is easy to understand how this belief originated since we all know what it feels like to be under stress. We can all recall the symptoms we feel when we are anxious. We jump at strange sounds in the night, our flesh crawling with goose bumps. On an airplane during a storm we white-knuckle the arms of our seats, as our sweat runs cold and our hearts beat faster. All these symptoms of anxiety, directly related to the stress of the moment, disappear quickly after the stressful moment is gone. Feeling anxious is part of being human, a universal feeling. It is not a disease. Anxiety disease differs from ordinary anxiousness in two ways: anxiety symptoms are so severe that they interfere with how we want to live, and they often occur without any apparent reason. Anxiety disease may or *may not* be related to stress. One thing is certain: removing the stress will *not* cure the disease.

Some people don't seek treatment simply because of who they are. Many sufferers are strong-willed, individualistic, and self-sufficient people. Their methods of handling problems in the past have been to meet them head-on with determination and perseverance until the problem is solved. They view seeking help as a sign of weakness or a crutch. While their head-on approach can be effective for many problems, it is useless against anxiety disease.

One of my patients, a highly venerated priest, was sure that he did not need help once his problem, anxiety disease, was identified. When he became so ill that he could not even preside at meetings, he agreed to take medication for a short time. The improvement was remarkable. Then, after two weeks he decided to try it on his own and ceased taking the medication. He flew off to a national meeting, but soon called me to say that his condition had worsened. We went through this cycle three times before he finally agreed to complete the full treatment plan. Exodus tells us that "God made the Pharoah obdurate." I thought for a while that my friend might need to be "plagued" all seven times before he saw the light.

Another reason for not getting help is often the nature of the symptoms. "Weird things are happening to me, really bizarre things. My body feels odd all over. It's embarrassing. I'm too ashamed to talk about it. Besides, no one would believe me anyway. Maybe I really am losing my mind."

One patient described his first episode of panic, which occurred during a meeting of the Board of Trustees of his bank. The meeting was friendly, but intense. In the middle of this session he suddenly felt an overwhelming need to get out quickly. He had no idea why and could not identify any danger, physical symptom, or logic. He just knew he had to get out of the room. He was farthest from the door and would have had to bolt right through the group to escape. Instead he just sat and trembled, sweated for a while, and then hurried off to the bathroom. After about ten minutes he felt better. He told this to no one for years, not until he was sure he wasn't having a "nervous breakdown" or "going crazy." He just hoped it wouldn't happen again, but ever since that episode he always sits near the door during meetings, just in case.

He saw a physician regularly for other reasons, but never mentioned this terrifying episode, and the doctor's questions never probed deeply enough to uncover it. A physician's standard questions usually don't stimulate any thoughtful responses. "Do you get depressed? Are you worried about anything? How are your nerves? Do you sleep okay? Are you irritable?" Most of them require only a simple yes or no answer. We doctors are just beginning to learn how to invite you to voice your real feelings, beginning with comments like "Let's talk about your feelings," or "tell me about the last time you felt. . . ." We are just learning, though, so you may need to help us.

In fact, some of the blame for people's reticence to seek treatment can be placed right in the lap of the health profession itself. Too often too many doctors say or imply with great impatience, "It's all in your head." Most doctors are trained to seek out diseases they can see or locate and attack with a pill or a knife. Some gynecologists, when looking and not finding a disease of the female reproductive system, will conclude that no disease exists or that the problem lies elsewhere. "You need to see a different specialist," they may offer. Yet such comments frequently seem to be attributing the blame to the patient's imagination.

Physicians whose practice is limited to particular diseases, systems, or treatment methods, look for the disease that fits into their specialty area. Lack of familiarity with the prevalence and differing forms and faces of anxiety disease can clearly add to the problem of making a correct diagnosis.

Another obstacle is that many people believe that treatment won't help them anyway. "How can medicines affect how I think or feel? And if they can, I don't want to take them. That sounds like drugs. I'll get hooked and never be able to get off them. Or else I'll end up on a couch talking about my childhood at $100 an hour. No, thank you! I'll handle this my way."

One of the many good things happening in modern science is that recently many people are becoming wary of drugs—any kind of drug. The dangers of narcotics and the so-called recreational drugs have been well publicized. But every prescription drug also carries dangers. More and more people are asking questions about side effects, mixing one drug with another or with alcohol, and asking what the dangers are of taking too much or too little.

This is a very healthy practice. However, it makes sense to balance the dangers of using prescription drugs against the dangers of not using them. Totally avoiding treatment out of fear of drugs, without weighing the potential risks and advantages, doesn't make sense. It can be self-defeating and is simply not a healthy way to live.

One of my patients, a middle-aged businesswoman, delayed getting help for her anxiety disease for more than a year because her oldest son was in jail on drug charges. She wasn't "taking any chances." When she finally did agree to accept treatment, however, she needed to take medications for only seven or eight weeks.

Another reason why so many people remain untreated is the very nature of the disease. Panic attacks, one of the most frequent forms of anxiety disease, are often complicated by agoraphobia, an imprisoning fear of open spaces, or, in some cases, of even leaving home. How can you get treatment if you can't leave your house? Psychiatrists don't make home calls. Most family physicians and general practitioners do, but only for clearcut medical reasons—probably not for the patient who says, "I just don't feel like going out."

Most people, more than 75%, with anxiety disease, don't seek help because of a fear of being misunderstood, a sense of futility about treatment, or a fear of using drugs. These are very understandable reasons. Who wants to pay a fee, only to be insulted by the attitude, "You don't have a *real* disease." Why look for help when we don't believe treatment will work?

If you or a loved one has anxiety disease, these are disturbing questions. But there is good news!

YOU ARE NOT ALONE

One out of ten people has an anxiety disease. That may not sound like good news, and certainly sounds insensitive. But there is some comfort in knowing that you are not alone, and that there are literally millions of other people experiencing this same debilitating disease. It's even more comforting to know that relief exists.

It is a great comfort to talk with someone else, someone who has also had strange and even frightening feelings, unusual symptoms, and perhaps has also been looked at askance by family, friends, or doctors. There is something mysterious, but absolutely dependable, about the relief that comes from discussing your experiences with another person who has had similar occurrences, be it a friend, professional, or hairdresser. Since numerous people have anxiety disease, it shouldn't be too difficult to find a fellow sufferer who can empathize with you.

Of course, just having more people around with anxiety disease wouldn't help a bit if they were unknown and isolated. That brings us to the second chunk of comforting news.

OUT OF THE CLOSET

What a miserable, lonely feeling it is to know that you have a physical ailment, one that absolutely forbids you to live the kind of life you want, and know that it is not socially acceptable to discuss it. It must feel akin to knowing that you had syphilis before there were antibiotics. You feel as though you can't discuss it openly, and that people would say you should have been more careful. So it is with anxiety disease. People wonder, "How can I allow myself the weakness of a nervous breakdown, or be so weak as to let my nerves get me down?"

Until now it was often better not to mention your anxiety disease symptoms rather than tolerate scornful glances, disapproving looks, and snide remarks. Many people have lived an even bigger lie, often unwittingly, blaming all of their symptoms on another physical disease such as a heart condition, arthritis, or rheumatism. Often these diagnoses have been aided and abetted, also unwittingly, by physicians. But even when you know better, it has always been much more acceptable to discuss your heart, bone, or muscle problem then your "nerves."

Fortunately, today all of this is changing. People are beginning to "admit" that they suffer from an anxiety disease. Notice, though, that there is still an element of guilt. No one "admits" to having heart disease or arthritis.

I first saw Mr. Stewart as a patient when he was in his late sixties. A retired state bureaucrat, he was healthy and happy until about six months before when he began to experience increasing fatigue. Concerned, he went to his family doctor who did the appropriate history, physical examination, and tests and concluded that Mr. Stewart had anxiety disease. He discussed this with his patient and prescribed antianxiety medication. Mr. Stewart was no incensed by the diagnosis that he did not fill the prescription and made an appointment to see me, also a family physician, instead.

After I completed my work-up, I offered Mr. Stewart a prescription for his fatigue. He pointedly avoided asking me for my diagnosis and agreed to take the medication for "my tiredness." One month and three visits later we were able to discuss Mr. Stewart's anxiety disease by name, although he was still reluctant to use the words and preferred instead to talk about "my tiredness."

For some, anxiety disease is not altogether out of the closet, but the door is open a crack, and fresh, honest, caring air is blowing through.

DOCTORS ARE LEARNING

Anxiety diseases are out of the closet partly due to the array of new discoveries and treatments now available. However, most doctors in practice today were trained before modern drugs for anxiety disease were thoroughly tested and accepted. Some of the current thinking runs directly contrary to what they were taught in medical school. Many have had patients who had bad experiences with earlier drug prototypes. Other physicians are so worried about the possible addicting properties of antianxiety drugs that they refuse to prescribe them at all. Added to this is the simple fact that doctors are a cautious lot. This, I believe, is a good thing.

While many doctors are not yet familiar with newer diagnostic and treatment methods, many do keep abreast. The medical journals have published hundreds of articles on these subjects within the past five years. National meetings of primary care groups, the American Academy of Family Physicians, the American Osteopathic Association, and the College of Physicians have had frequent presentations on the new diagnostic and therapeutic methods of dealing with anxiety diseases. I have personally participated in a score of these meetings which involved a total of more than 10,000 primary care physicians—family doctors, general practitioners, primary care internists—and psychiatrists.

However, good news does travel slowly. If you don't know your doctor well, or don't know how well she or he is versed in the modern approach to anxiety disease, it is a good idea to ask key questions before spending much time and money.

THE RIGHT DIAGNOSIS

Many basic diagnoses are very easy to make. Anyone can tell what's wrong when a leg is bent in the wrong direction or an arrow is sticking out of a person's chest. Other diagnoses are easy to make based on simple tests, such as a blood test for diabetes, a urine test for pregnancy, or an x-ray for a cracked bone.

Unfortunately, there are no blood tests, x-rays, or scans that can spot any particular anxiety disease. Tests may be helpful in ruling out other diseases that could be causing the same symptoms or in deciding how much of the chest pain is from heart disease, how much from anxiety, and how much from the arrow sticking out of the patient's chest.

Some anxiety diseases can be diagnosed by the person's clinical history, the story of what is happening. For example, a phobia is defined as a persistent, excessive, and unreasonable fear that leads an individual to avoid the precipitating stimulus. If the phobia interferes with the individual's life, it is considered to be an anxiety disease for which the person might want treatment.

Mrs. Johnson has a snake phobia. She has severe anxiety symptoms every time she sees a snake, even on television. Fortunately, she lives in a high-rise in mid-Manhattan, and her office is in one of the World Trade towers. She can plan her life to avoid ever glimpsing a snake. She does have a phobia, but only as an idiosyncrasy of her personality, not as an anxiety disease requiring treatment. However, if Mrs. Johnson's employer offered her the opportunity to manage a new plant in Snake River, Wyoming, her phobia might affect her decision. Then it would be considered an anxiety disease and she might wish to seek appropriate treatment.

Suppose a man is subject to severe midchest pains, sweating, and shortness of breath. Perhaps this man is also a smoker, is overweight, with a family history of heart disease, and has no arrow sticking out of his chest. Deciding whether these symptoms are being caused by heart disease, anxiety, or by a combination of both, is difficult but extremely important to determine. If this same man has just suffered the death of his wife, then are the chest pains part of the "heartache" of normal grief, an anxiety disease, a heart disease, or a combination of all three?

Despite the presence of these complexities, we can now make precise and certain diagnoses. In the early 1970s the American Psychiatric Association developed the *Diagnostic and Statistical Manual of Mental Disorders (DSM)*. Now in its third form revised, the *DSM III-R* has become a vital diagnostic tool. It not only provides a specific description of each of the anxiety diseases, it also includes information about how each disease develops. But most useful of all is a set of criteria that must be met for the verification of each particular diagnosis. So now it is possible, after the background information has been gathered, including the story of how the sickness started and other general health information, for a physician to make an exact diagnosis.

A precise diagnosis, a few years ago, would have been quite irrelevant, since treatment was hit or miss and the available drugs were mostly ineffective. All of that has changed drastically, which makes for the wonderful news that treatment works, provided the right treatment is matched with the right diagnosis.

TREATMENT WORKS

Most of us grew up in a time when anxiety disease, if diagnosed at all, was called something else, and the treatment for whatever it was called didn't do much good. The mainstay of treatment was counseling, usually focusing on past conflicts and stress, and simply learning how to cope with life better. The medications used were bromides first, then barbiturates, and, more recently, meprobamate (Miltown, Equanil). These drugs produced a calming effect, and even put people to sleep, but were not able to relieve their underlying anxiety, and could not help a person recover from the basic disease. If fact, serious side effects were later discovered. The bromides tended to accumulate and cause a chronic brain disease. Barbiturates are potentially addictive drugs and, in conjunction with alcohol, could prove lethal. Meprobamate has motor system side effects including loss of balance, slurred speech, and drowsiness. It is a sedative with no success as an antianxiety drug.

Over the years I have treated many, many people suffering from different forms of anxiety disease. In the past, the most the patient and I could achieve was some relief of the acute symptoms and some help in learning how to live with a chronic disease. Sometimes I could help other members of the family understand the diseases, but often I could not.

Now all of that has changed and actually has been reversed, thanks to new medications, especially the benzodiazepines such as Ativan, Xanax, and Valium, and the discoveries of how they affect the chemistry of the brain. For certain kinds of anxiety disease, medication is the primary form of treatment, with some help from counseling. For most kinds of anxiety disease, treatment consists of a combination of both methods. For a small number of diseases treatment consists of either one or the other. Present medications are wonderfully effective. It is not even necessary for a person to believe in the medications for them to work. I have had many patients who objected to taking drugs for anxiety disease because they didn't believe they really had it. They agreed to take the medication only because I insisted and only became believers when their symptoms disappeared.

Present treatment for anxiety disease is effective and can be quite safe, but requires careful monitoring by someone with knowledge and skill in these forms of treatment.

ANXIOUSNESS

We all have anxious moments and anxious times. It is part of being human. We worry about what people think of us, about mistakes we have made, about what will happen in the future, and who will find out about our mistakes. Often, we worry about security, health, money, protection, family, or jobs. Since we all really know that life is fragile, that all security is transient, and that we are likely to keep on making mistakes, we realize that there are plenty of reasons for us to feel anxious.

It all begins very early in our careers as humans. Perhaps the first recollection, if you think about it, was being caught with your hand in the pretzel jar. How did you cope with that moment of terror and raw anxiety? Blame it on someone else: "Sis made me do it." Denial: "I only wanted to count the pretzels." Flee: Hide under the table. Get sick: Moan with a terrible bellyache. Or if all else fails, admit it and ask to be forgiven.

All of this is part of the learning process, the multiple-choice questions that we all face in choosing how to deal with our own anxiousness. The intense discomfort of being anxious also affects our choices of how we live, and how we learn to avoid that pain. Are the pretzels really worth the price?

As we grow up and life becomes more complicated, we find ourselves in situations over which we have little or no control. Will our team win? Will my sweetheart say yes? Will our baby be okay? Will our kids stay off drugs? Will my company be sold? Will I be able to eat pretzels with false teeth?

We handle the reactions in the ways we have gradually learned over a lifetime. We may try to deny or distract ourselves by keeping busy, or fleeing, or accepting a situation and learning to live with it, or sharing our feelings with a friend or health professional. The different ways of handling our anxieties are almost as numerous as the situations that make us anxious.

Regardless of the causes, we have learned to recognize the physical symptoms that accompany sudden anxiety. As we noted earlier, these probably include palpitations (rapid or irregular heartbeat), sweating, trembling, a sense of fear that something terrible is happening, and shortness of breath. The symptoms might also include pain in the stomach, diarrhea, an urge to urinate, dizziness, weak knees, and dry mouth. The symptoms we experience when anxiety is prolonged often consist of a variety of these acute symptoms. In time most people come to recognize their own pattern of response to stress.

Once we recognize our symptoms of anxiety, we automatically use the coping methods that have worked best for us in the past. We may or may not have caused the anxious situation, but it is up to us to deal with it. No one else is likely to be able to do it for us. It is our responsibility. In a sense it is our own fault if it takes a long time to get ourselves under control.

ANXIETY DISEASE

That is how we recognize, feel, and deal with everyday anxiousness. Anxiety disease is a far more serious problem, but it often begins with the same set of symptoms. When this happens, how is the body supposed to know when anxiousness stops and the disease begins? Since that transition can be very sneaky, it is only natural for the sufferers to feel that if they are not getting over their symptoms, it is because they aren't coping well. In other words, it is their own fault! "I just have to get myself together, try again, pray harder, think positively, or ignore these symptoms and everything will be okay."

This is often how the self-accusations, the feelings of personal inadequacy and failure begin. At this point it would be exhilarating to have a friend say, "Hey, it's not your fault. You have a serious, disabling problem, but you didn't want it, you didn't do it. It's not your fault."

Unfortunately, this doesn't happen often. It's not because you don't have faithful friends or caring loved ones. The truth is that they have the same background as you do, and they may not be able to see the difference between coping with real anxiousness and anxiety disease any better than you can. So they offer you the same pep talk you give yourself, "Don't worry, be happy. Do like I do, keep busy, think of something else, pretend everything is okay and it will be."

And so the destructive cycle begins. Anxiety diseases are diseases of fear and doubt. When this is reinforced by your own fears and the fears and doubts of family and friends, the fear is compounded with guilt. Sometimes the whole cycle is given another twist by an unknowing or insensitive physician who suggests, "You don't have a real disease. All your tests and examinations are normal. It's all in your mind. It's just your nerves."

I am happy to say that for all of the fears and doubts whirling in your mind, for the misery and the unanswered questions, "What's happening to me? What's wrong with me? Am I losing my mind? What have I done wrong?" there are now solid answers that will help you heal.

We now know that *anxiety disease is not your fault*. We know that while stress may be a factor in precipitating anxiety disease, it can start with chemical changes in the body over which you have no control. Just as people with diabetes or gout have no control over the symptoms of their diseases, neither do you.

You did not try to get this disease. You couldn't get it by yourself if you did try. You don't want it and you cannot wish it away. You can't even hide it in the closet for long.

Anxiety disease is an actual disease with real and unpleasant symptoms. It's not all in your head. It's not just your nerves. And most important of all, it is not your fault.

Ask the patient, not the doctor, where the
pain is.

Hindu Proverb

Chapter 2

Three Faces of Anxiety Disease

When I was a medical student, an older physician told me, "You can learn most if you listen to your patient." It sounded trite at the time, but 40 years of practicing medicine in the same small town has given me a more incisive perspective on many things.

"Listen to your patient." For many people I have been the family doctor for three generations, and often the only doctor they've ever known. I've made calls to their homes, watched and helped them grow and change, often becoming an ex officio member of their families. I've seen their patterns of health and sickness, and I know how they live their lives, how they manage stress, and how they cope. We have shared our thoughts, beliefs, and values.

From them, I've learned to listen. I have a textbook that describes a typical panic attack as an episode that develops suddenly, includes at least four of thirteen possible symptoms, and subsides in ten minutes. It is a valuable definition, but it is not the same as sitting with a patient, perhaps touching a hand, and listening to the description of the recent attack: the urgent need, the stark terror, the sudden overwhelming fear, pounding heart, panting breath, trembling, and sweating.

So that you can listen too, I will introduce you to three people who suffered from anxiety disease. In several instances you will also note that they suffered from the clumsiness of their physician, me, in diagnosing and treating their disease. These episodes are included not by way of confession, but as illustrations of the state of knowledge and my own limits at the time.

I visited each of these people in their homes and asked permission to include their stories in this book. I changed their personal data to protect their privacy, but the stories are real, and all of the important events did happen. All three not only gave their permission, but were eager to help, hoping that their stories might help others.

RUTH

About four years ago, Ruth came to see me. She had been my patient for twenty-five years, and for twenty-five years she had had an annual physical examination every August. Since she was healthy, happy, active, self-assured, and generally delightful, I rarely saw her at any other time. But when she came in April, I knew something was wrong. So did Ruth, but she didn't know what.

Sitting there she had a far away look in her eyes: "I just don't feel well." I listened, but I didn't hear words that helped me. She felt "a kind of achiness all over," "a sort of dizziness," and "just not right." Perhaps she couldn't describe her symptoms clearly because she was not used to being sick and didn't know the usual patient terms. Perhaps. I did hear that she felt bad and was unhappy about it.

I examined her and found nothing obviously wrong. She had lost some weight, about seven pounds, which was unusual since she had always maintained a near ideal weight. With other patients I might have adopted a wait-and-see attitude, but Ruth had been so healthy and free of complaints, that I was concerned there was a problem I just couldn't find. I ran a whole battery of tests looking for any hint of inflammation, anemia, endocrine or electrolyte imbalance. Nothing. Everything was normal.

Yet her symptoms got worse over the next few weeks. She was able to describe them better, but it didn't help me very much. She had headaches, often in the back of her head, but sometimes in the front. Sometimes there was a muscular stiffness in the back of her neck. Her joints hurt, especially her knees and lower back, but sometimes her shoulders, too. The dizziness was worse, but she didn't feel as if she would pass out. The skin on her back and legs tingled, feeling hot and cold.

I tried blaming her symptoms on menopause since she was almost fifty and her menstrual periods had nearly stopped. She had slight heat flashes and some irritability, but neither of us believed me and the usual remedies made no difference in her symptoms.

I ran more tests. This time I included a chest x-ray, electrocardiogram, breathing tests, back x-ray, more blood work, and stool and urine examinations. I even ran a CAT scan, thinking perhaps a brain tumor? Nothing. All the tests returned normal.

But my patient was not. She was clearly miserable. For all of these tests and examinations she had been in my office at least once, sometimes twice weekly. I used some of that time to listen, to explore her life and feelings.

She felt sick and she was worried about what was causing it. Moreover, her life was free of unusual stress. She was happy with her life, her husband, and her children. She and Alan, married for twenty years, had a loving, comfortable relationship. They enjoyed good sexual relations, though she hadn't been very interested lately. Although she was teaching when I first met her, she retired after her second baby to stay home and raise her family. The children, both delivered by me, were now in their late teens and well past their difficult periods. She and Alan were delighted with the direction their lives were taking. She didn't miss teaching, but worked part time in a boutique just to be around people. She was active in her church and several organizations. Her social life was full and she had many friends.

All in all, Ruth was a happy, well-adjusted woman. But she was sick, and I hadn't found out what was wrong with her. I suggested referral to another specialty, and she asked, pointedly, which one—rheumatology, orthopedics, psychiatry, neurology, gynecology? I didn't have an answer for that, and decided to run another battery of blood tests. Ruth agreed. This time her tests showed small, but definite signs of overactive thyroid disease. Hyperthyroidism could cause all of her symptoms, although I had no idea why her previous tests were normal or why these showed such a slight increase. I was relieved to have an explanation, and knew we should be able to control the disease.

I was also pleased with the timing of the diagnosis. I was about to leave for a six-month sabbatical, and both Ruth and I were concerned about her care. I arranged for her to have a consultation with an endocrinologist, who agreed to treat her in my absence. The endocrinologist was also perplexed by the disparity between the length and severity of Ruth's symptoms and the slight change in her blood tests.

Ruth was among the first of my patients when I returned from sabbatical. I had hoped to find her well and happy, but instead she was gaunt, having lost another eight pounds. She was jumpy, irritable, and thoroughly frightened, convinced that she had all sorts of morbid diseases, from cancer to multiple sclerosis or AIDS, which we just hadn't found.

While I was away she had continued treatment with the endocrinologist. When her blood tests returned to normal but her symptoms didn't improve, her endocrinologist changed the diagnosis to hyperdynamic beta-adrenergic circulatory state. This is the name given to a cluster of symptoms characterized by the overactivity of the autonomic nervous system, which controls the function of the internal organs. Overactivity can cause dizziness, aching, palpitations, hot and cold feelings, fatigue, and a host of other miseries.

For this she was treated with beta blockers, drugs specifically designed to counteract overactivity of the autonomic nervous system. Although these drugs are very effective, they sometimes have side effects of fatigue and depression. Ruth experienced both of these, with no improvement in her basic condition. Her endocrinologist changed the prescription around, still trying to find the best dosage. Meanwhile, Ruth's condition remained the same.

"Just yesterday," she recounted, trembling, "I was in the grocery store. It was crowded as always on Thursdays, and I really hadn't felt right all day. But I got the things I needed and stood in the check-out line, when it happened again. Suddenly I felt hot and cold all over, like I might pass out or even go crazy. I can't really describe it, but I knew I just had to get out of there. I shoved my cart to the side and practically ran out of the store. It was awful, and it almost happened again in the waiting room. What's happening to me? Am I losing my mind?"

As I listened the pieces suddenly fell into place. Though somewhat belatedly, I knew I had answers. While on sabbatical I had done some special work in the field of anxiety. It was time well spent. It seemed startlingly clear to me that Ruth had been suffering from anxiety disease all along.

Her grocery store episode was a perfect description of a panic attack. Her symptoms often occurred as a group of "little panic attacks." I call them "little panic attacks" because they don't include all of the textbook symptoms, but to someone who has them, there's nothing little about them at all.

Between these attacks she became more and more anxious that she would have another. She was especially fearful that she would have one while away from her home and family. She consequently stayed home more and more. Finally, she even quit her job and stopped attending church and meetings. The only friends she saw were those who came to her. She stopped going out for dinner, although it had long been a favorite activity. The one time she tried, she became so afraid of having another attack that she had to leave and sit in the car.

I explained my diagnosis and told her there was a cure. Ruth seemed uncertain. She was unfamiliar with the terms anxiety disease, panic attacks, and agoraphobia, pointing out again and again that she had no anxiety or stress in her life until all of these symptoms started. Anxiety disease, I told her, is not always precipitated by stress. Sometimes it just happens, apparently from some chemical changes in the body that we can't yet detect with a laboratory test. Ruth was skeptical, and who could blame her after all the time she spent taking tests and all of the false starts?

ROBERT

When Robert came to my office, he was clearly distressed, having called three times to check his appointment time. Then he arrived thirty minutes early. He paced the waiting room ceaselessly, using the bathroom twice before his appointment.

I had not seen Robert in nearly three years. He greeted me with a troubled look and a clammy handshake. He couldn't sit still, and his lean body was restless, constantly moving. His jaws twitched as the words tumbled out.

"Doc, I got this bad pain right here in my heart on Saturday night. I thought it was just gas, but it kept getting worse, so I went to the emergency room. They did all kinds of tests and said it was 'just my nerves.' I don't believe that. My nerves are fine. What have I got to be nervous about, anyway? So I came to you to find out what's really wrong."

I examined him and listened. He was thirty-seven years old, and except for college, had lived in this county all his life. He was a certified public accountant with a reputation for excellence. He clearly loved his work.

He also clearly loved his wife, Elaine. They had been happily married for ten years without any serious quarrels or problems. She kept their home in the Pennsylvania Dutch tradition—everything in the house is cleaned regularly whether it needs it or not, and the porch, sidewalk, and street, are swept daily. She worked part time as a bookkeeper. And she idolized Robert. They had no children: "It just didn't happen." Leisure time was spent together taking care of their home, attending community events, and visiting friends. Although they were members of the Methodist church, they were not active.

Robert had been generally healthy, although he had an appendectomy when he was seventeen. In college he had several episodes of breathing difficulty, which were "like asthma without the wheezing." Each time, the college dispensary gave him some medication and the attack went away. He'd only experienced these episodes a few times since school and none were severe.

When his mother died of cancer in her early fifties, his father suffered a nervous breakdown. Robert was not sure exactly what that meant, but blamed it on a grief reaction, and explained that he "never really got over it."

We talked about his experience last Saturday night. He and Elaine were playing bridge with friends when pain took hold of the front of his chest. At first he thought it was gas, but when it didn't go away they took him to the hospital emergency room. The doctor told him that his blood pressure was borderline normal, and his pulse was a little fast with a slight irregularity. His electrocardiogram, chest x-ray, and blood tests were also normal. The doctor told him it must be a stress reaction and suggested he go home and rest. He offered a prescription for a "nerve pill," but Robert refused.

I examined him carefully, looking for some sign of heart disease, but found none. His pulse was rapid with an occasional extra beat, but except for that and his restlessness and apprehension, his examination was entirely normal. I considered the possibility of overactive thyroid disease, which can cause rapid and irregular heartbeat, nervousness, sweating, apprehension, and even chest pain. However, the sudden onset and normal examination made that unlikely.

Much more likely was some form of anxiety disease. Although I wanted to observe him over a period of time, I offered him a medication that would give some immediate relief. I also hoped it would help convince him that his symptoms really were due to anxiety.

"No thanks," he said, assuring me that if it really were anxiety, he would have plenty of time to relax and "get himself together" over the upcoming Thanksgiving weekend.

I carefully explained that anxiety disease may come from chemical changes within his body, not from a failure to "get himself together," and that it was unlikely he could "will" it to go away.

He politely but firmly refused, so I invited him to call me if he had any further trouble.

He called later that same day, still shaken from an episode he had just experienced. While watching television he unaccountably had begun to sweat and feel short of breath. No chest pain this time, but he felt that he might have collapsed or even died. I explained that these are signs of the anxiety disease and again suggested medication. He hardly remembered that we discussed medication before. That wasn't surprising since a common problem in anxiety disease is the inability to concentrate and remember. He was still quite determined, however, not to take any "nerve" medicine.

Robert came to see me first thing Monday morning. Miserable and frightened, he was certain that something was drastically wrong with his body. Thanksgiving Day was especially bad. He had experienced chest pain and shortness of breath several times, though this time without the sweating. He'd also had diarrhea, and was just too uncomfortable to sit through a whole meal.

Since the next day proved better, he thought maybe the whole episode was no more than a touch of virus. But over the weekend everything got worse, compounded by a growing restlessness. Now even his sleeping was affected; he had trouble falling asleep and when he finally did, he awakened frequently. He simply could not eat.

I examined him again, and found nothing new. I repeated his electrocardiogram and did a simple breathing test, a vital capacity measurement. I thought both of these might help reassure him, and the breathing test would tell me if he were unable to get enough air into his lungs. Both tests were normal.

Elaine accompanied him this time, so the three of us discussed what was happening to Robert. Elaine was worried. Over the past two months she said Robert had been somewhat irritable, which was highly unusual for him. At first she blamed that and their decreased sexual activity on job pressures. When he began having physical complaints, chest discomforts, diarrhea, gas, and indigestion, she wanted him to see a doctor. Each time he refused angrily, blaming each episode on a particular food or some activity.

I believed Robert was suffering from the disease called panic attack.

PAUL

Paul came right to the point. "Doc, you gotta help me—I think I'm losing my mind."

I'd known Paul a long time. We had met in the high school kitchen when we were both flipping pancakes for a fund-raising breakfast for the school band. Eventually he came to see me for a routine physical. He had been my patient ever since.

At that first physical examination I found him to be quite healthy, although he had experienced several episodes of illness in the previous year. He'd had two attacks of diarrhea and upset stomach, possibly due to a virus, and one attack of sudden shortness of breath, for which he was seen in the hospital emergency room. No cause was found, but his breathing returned to normal before the tests were finished and he'd had no further attacks. He had a family history of diabetes (his mother) and high blood pressure (both parents).

Paul and Edna fell in love and married when both were thirty-six, a first marriage for each. Within a year, Paul's younger sister died leaving two preschool-age children. Paul and Edna immediately adopted both of them. It's a decision I would have advised against, considering all of the factors. Happily, they didn't ask my advice, and their decision turned out to be a beautiful one for all of them. In three years they added a child of their own. By this time I was treating Paul for both diabetes and high blood pressure. The diabetes was easily controlled by diet, and the high blood pressure with medication.

Except for the usual illnesses and mishaps of children, life continued happily and healthfully for Paul and his family. Over the years Paul continued to have occasional episodes of illness—gastrointestinal upsets, chest discomfort, sometimes just vague complaints that he couldn't quite explain. They were definitely unrelated to either his diabetes or high blood pressure, although he worried that they were. His symptoms never persisted and I could never discern a pattern. Sometimes an attack seemed to be related to some new problem at work, but more often they were not.

Now, at the age of fifty-eight, Paul was back in my office, urgently asking my help for an entirely new problem.

He had been driving home from work on a country road. In the dark, he had missed a turn and hit a tree. He was admitted to the hospital for multiple injuries. Fortunately, he had been wearing a seat belt, so the injuries turned out to be minor. However, he had been in the hospital for three days. Thoughts of what had happened, and the awful things that could have happened, haunted him. Suppose his family had been with him? Suppose he had swerved left instead of right and hit another family?

During those three days of thinking Paul finally admitted to himself that he hadn't really fallen asleep at the wheel. He just wasn't thinking about driving. His mind was elsewhere—out of focus, maybe out of control.

With obvious difficulty Paul then described what he had been going through during the previous few months. At first he thought he was just distracted because of pressure at work. He couldn't seem to keep his mind focused. Then he realized he was forgetting things—too many things. He had forgotten Edna's birthday, which had never happened before. Work wasn't going well. He worked longer hours to try to be more productive, but that didn't seem to help much. He knew he wasn't as creative as he had been, that he couldn't seem to come up with the fresh ideas he had in the past. He blamed all of this on his age at first, but he worried more and more that there was some other reason—Alzheimer's disease, probably. And the more he worried, the less he could concentrate. The three days of nothing else to think about in the hospital had brought him to the conclusion he had been trying so hard to avoid—his mind was going.

I was alarmed too. The symptom pattern could be the start of Alzheimer's or some other form of organic brain disease. I immediately did a thorough neurological exam, but found nothing abnormal. That didn't mean much, though. I wouldn't expect to find gross neurological or mental changes early in Alzheimer's disease. But Paul already seemed somewhat relieved. Perhaps this was simply because he had unburdened himself of his gnawing fear.

I asked him to allow me to arrange a consultation with a psychologist for a thorough battery of psychological tests and he readily agreed. The tests showed no hint of brain disease of any kind. They did reflect some evidence of his worrying, but nothing considered abnormal under the circumstances.

Paul was enormously relieved, although he had actually begun to feel more confident even before the test results were reported. The next time I saw him, again socially, was at the annual high school pancake breakfast. He said he was feeling like his old self again—and Edna beamed her agreement.

Almost a year later, Paul was in my office with a new problem of severe night sweats. At least twice each night he awakened with such drenching sweat that he had to change pajamas and occasionally the sheets.

This was an alarming symptom. The most likely cause was an infection like tuberculosis, a lymphatic cancer such as lymphoma, or even malaria, since at one time he had been in the tropics. I did a complete physical examination including x-rays and blood tests. All was normal. Paul said he thought it was his blood pressure medication, so he had stopped taking it, but found no improvement.

By the time the studies were complete, Paul was having attacks of diarrhea, abdominal cramps, and unexplained episodes of shortness of breath. He was irritable at home and at work and always felt tired.

Through all this I was aware of his continuing, smoldering anger. When I asked about it, he said, "What have I got to be angry about?" I probed gently, and he finally confided to me that he was having problems at work. A successful businessman, he had moved well within his company. His performance evaluations and promotions had been good. But his company had recently changed its personnel policy for people at his level. It was suggested that he consider an early retirement at age sixty, just a few months away. He had rejected the idea because he really liked his job. But now the pressure was increasing. He knew that if he did not volunteer gracefully, he would be forced out.

Paul and I talked about the situation for several weeks and he finally decided to accept the offer. His only real concern now was his survival. He continued to feel worse.

Paul's tests and examinations were still normal. I considered the whole pattern of his symptoms—the episodes of gastrointestinal upset, the attacks of shortness of breath, the time he thought he was losing his mind, the irritability and anger (unusual for easygoing Paul), and the soaking night sweats. While his work situation was enough to produce anxiety, his symptoms had really begun before that crisis. I knew that Paul was suffering from generalized anxiety disorder.

In typical Paul fashion, he flatly refused to seek a second opinion even though he was equally convinced that my diagnosis was wrong. Edna continued to be supportive, but she, too, was unconvinced about the diagnosis, certain that all of Paul's problems were somehow related to retirement. Almost in desperation, he agreed to try some medication.

When he returned in two weeks he was smiling broadly, happy to report that the night sweats were less severe and many of his other symptoms were greatly improved, though he still had some very bad days.

It would seem that this story should have had an easy, happy ending. Paul continued his medication and continued to improve, though not steadily, for the next two months. Then, gradually his feeling of fatigue increased. He blamed it on awakening too early, at four or five every morning. He also gained ten pounds and admitted that he had abandoned his dietary precautions and his blood pressure medication. "Doc, I just don't give a damn."

His anxiety disease had become complicated by symptoms of depression.

Paul didn't like this diagnosis either. "Why should I be depressed? I don't have to work. I have no money worries. The kids are great. I don't even have to worry about the twenty-four people who used to work for me. The only thing to be depressed about is that I don't feel well."

I suggested that his "I don't give a damn" feeling might be related to his early retirement. That would certainly be natural enough, but since it had been getting worse for several months, perhaps he needed some help.

Like anxiety, depression is often both physiological and psychological in origin. Treatment requires both counseling and medication. Finally he agreed to take an additional antidepressant medication.

CONCLUSION

For now we leave these stories incomplete. I chose them because I learned a great deal from them and believe that they have much to teach us all.

Each patient had an anxiety disease. Each was under my care for a prolonged period of time. Each had a strong, individualistic personality. But there are actually more differences among these people than similarities.

Their backgrounds, circumstances, and families were quite distinct from each other. Anxiety disease attacked each one differently and each experienced different symptoms. Even their reactions to illness were individual: Ruth was mystified; Robert was sure it was something else.

Paul's response was mixed. He was glad to believe he did not have

Alzheimer's disease, accepted the diagnosis of anxiety disease only after he improved, and completely denied that he was depressed.

Finding the correct diagnosis depended on understanding each patient as a whole person. Physical examinations and laboratory testing were helpful to prove that they didn't have something else. But the true diagnosis came from listening to them, their histories, symptoms and responses to illness, and also to their families.

Hippocrates said he diagnosed "by paying attention to what was common to every and particular to each case; to the patient . . . to the habits of life and occupation of each patient; to his speech, conduct, silences, thoughts, sleep, wakefulness, and dreams—their content and incidence; to his pickings and scratchings, tears, stools, urine, spit, and vomit."

The treatment also depends on understanding the whole person. Beliefs, values, and attitudes toward the various kinds of therapy and the therapist have much to do with its effectiveness.

Most people will only follow advice that makes sense to them, and conforms to their beliefs. Most people no longer accept the role of their predecessors two generations ago who nodded submissively, "You're the doctor." "Whatever you say, Doc."

I believe that this is a healthy change in an era when our treatments are potent enough to do miracles, but can also wreak havoc on mind and body. Patients need to ask hard questions. The treatment process should be a joint venture because so much depends directly on the trust relationship between patient and would-be healer. While that relationship is always important, it is absolutely essential in anxiety disease.

If we do not listen to our patients, we will not find the true diagnosis, nor will our patients listen to us when we suggest treatment.

rse has big head. Let him worry.
Anonymous

hapter 3

nxiety Is the Spouse of Life

ormal Anxiety and Anxiety Diseases

To live means to experience anxiety. Life is filled with uncertainty, and whenever there is uncertainty, there is also anxiousness. Anxiousness is not an evil to shun nor a hazard to avert; it is one of the discomforts of living a fuller life, like sweating and shortness of breath after a two-mile run or sexual intercourse.

If we adopt freedom from anxiousness as a life goal, then we must also accept sameness, monotony, uniformity, and mediocrity. Even then there will be some anxiety, and some worry that the unknown will deter us from our chosen road to nowhere. A fuller, richer, more daring life means more anxiety, and more anxiousness. It is the price of venturing into the unknown, of reaching out to others, and even of reaching inward to understand ourselves.

We all know what it's like to feel anxious. We have all experienced knotted stomachs, the trembling, nervousness, and sweating. It is part of our common experience, part of being human. It is important for us to realize that everyone experiences these same feelings, and it's not a weird quirk of our own.

We have all had sudden frights and keenly remember the physical discomforts that go along with them. For example, let's imagine that we are passengers in a car speeding along a two-lane highway approaching the top of a hill when suddenly we see an eighteen wheeler coming over the hill in our lane. A lot of things happen to us quickly, while the driver is busy braking, steering, cursing or praying, and likely unaware of any feelings until afterwards.

As passengers, we're likely to feel a sudden racing of our hearts. We may gasp or shout without meaning to. We may notice a lump in the throat that feels as though we couldn't swallow or as though we were trying to swallow over something. Our mouths might instantly turn so dry that we wouldn't be able to swallow anyway. If we were able to talk at all, our utterances would likely be tense, pressured, and inane. We might even lose control of our sphincters and defecate, urinate, or pass gas. We are likely to notice a cold, drenching sweat, especially over the upper half of the body. If we were to try to do anything such as crossing ourselves, we would notice that our hands shake uncontrollably.

Assuming that we survived this close call we probably would ask the driver to stop the car so that we could get out, but in doing so might notice that our knees were too shaky to hold us up. We probably would have difficulty making rational conversation. We might shout or sob while others might curse or be unable to speak at all. This is the kind of sudden anxiousness that we all have experienced in varying degrees.

These symptoms are the result of the body's automatic response to danger, popularly known as the "fight or flight" response. When a sudden danger is perceived by the senses—sight, hearing, smell, or touch, a signal is sent to the brain or central nervous system. It instantly activates the autonomic, or automatic, nervous system, which controls all of our internal organs, but over which we have no conscious control. One of the immediate responses is an outpouring of adrenalin from the adrenal glands. The sudden surge of adrenalin prepares us, in a primitive way, to take action: to fight the sabre-toothed tiger or to run away from it. Adrenalin quickens the heartbeat, increases blood pressure, and shuts down the blood supply to the other internal organs, such as the digestive organs, the bowel or the bladder where it is not needed during "fight or flight." Instead, it increases the blood supply to the muscles, the heart, and the lungs, which are the systems we need to run or to do battle.

This marvelous arrangement has helped humanity survive through the ages. Certainly it helps our driver's swift response to impending disaster by heightening awareness and response time. But for us, the passengers, it has done little but make us uncomfortable. We are prepared to run from the scene of an almost-accident, which makes little sense, or attack the danger, perhaps the other driver, which makes even less sense.

Fortunately, the system also has a shutdown mechanism. After the danger is past and we are rationally reconciled to it, there is no further outpouring of adrenalin and the adrenalin in circulation is dissipated or "used up." The symptoms may subside in a few minutes or last as long as an hour, depending on how severe the episode was and how strongly we responded to the threat.

We do have some degree of control over our response to danger through our conscious nervous system. If we are able to consider the situation reasonably, to recognize that the danger is past, and perhaps to gain some emotional support from spiritual inner strength or from each other, the symptoms will subside more quickly. On the other hand, if we dwell on the "might have beens," and visualize ourselves smashed against the windshield or contemplate a loved one being traumatized, our symptoms may continue for a long time. The symptoms might even come back to some degree whenever these thoughts recur.

This near-accident is an example of an episode that can easily cause an acute attack of anxiousness.

Even though the truck quickly returns to its own lane we may experience a few or all of these symptoms. These symptoms may also occur in a milder form when we experience small frights such as remembering that we left the house without turning off the iron or that we forgot to pay the insurance premium, or almost knocking over a shelf in an antique shop. All of these are examples of sudden anxiousness, and are clearly related to fear.

Other unexpected situations unrelated to fear can provoke the same response. If a woman comes home from work early, unexpectedly, and finds her husband in bed with the woman next door, all three will experience some sudden emotions. Most likely the wife's will be anger, but she will have the same symptoms as in the example of fear— preparation for fight or flight. This would include rapid pulse, rapid breathing, dry mouth, and tense muscles. The two in bed will also experience these symptoms including, no doubt, interference with sexual function. While the acute symptoms may lessen as each of them opts for a course of action, it is also probable that each will have some degree of continuing anxiety.

I encountered a young woman, named Jane, early in my practice, who was a chronic worrier. She had heart disease as a result of having contracted rheumatic fever when she was a teenager, and had many personal problems. She worried about her heart, about her daughter, and most of all, about the fact that she wasn't married to the man with whom she was living; they didn't want to give up the social security she would lose if she remarried. All of this resulted in various physical symptoms. She lived ten miles from my office and had very erratic transportation and no money, so she learned to phone whenever she had a new symptom. When it was apparent that the latest symptoms were related to anxiety, or worry, I would simply reassure her. If my wife or office nurse answered the phone, Jane would chat with them and feel equally reassured.

When I realized that her major worry was "living in sin," as she called it, I urged her to marry. Jane finally agreed to do so, but only if I made the arrangements, insisting that it must be in a church. Since she had no church affiliation they were married in our church, with her daughter as flower girl, my wife and I as witnesses, and our daughter as organist. The remarkable thing was that the symptoms disappeared almost magically, as did our daily telephone calls from Jane. Jane is an example of someone who suffered from chronic situational anxiety.

The symptoms of chronic long-term anxiety or worry are similar to acute symptoms but are less intense. There are often episodes of cold sweating associated with recurrent thoughts of guilt, or fear of being wrong. There may also be episodes of rapid heartbeating, fast breathing, or sighing. Speech patterns are often affected. Speech may seem pressured or hoarse, and sometimes there is stuttering or stammering. There is almost always interference with the thought process. These people have difficulty remembering, making decisions, or concentrating. The problem of not thinking clearly is compounded by their not really being able to perceive or understand what someone else is saying. This makes communication difficult for the chronic worrier or person with continuing anxiety. Trouble with communication means trouble with relationships, which adds fuel to the smoldering fires of anxiety.

Other physical symptoms of ongoing anxiety might include a need to urinate frequently because the bladder tenses and therefore, becomes smaller. It may also interfere with normal sexual function through a loss of interest in sex, or an inability to become physically aroused, or both. Some people have episodes of diarrhea, others constipation. Many people have difficulty eating while others seem to overeat, trying to placate their bodies. Most people have trouble sleeping, either having trouble getting to sleep or awakening often during the night.

As a result of these continuing symptoms, and the flow of adrenalin tensing the muscles, almost everyone with chronic worry or anxiety feels exhausted, usually without knowing why. The symptoms of chronic anxiety are bad enough, but not knowing why you are experiencing them makes them seem even worse.

TO WORRY IS HUMAN—SOMETIMES

Symptoms of acute anxiousness or worry, are all part of a person's normal response to life and is part of the price we pay for being human. We all worry, but it is ultimately a futile exercise and for the worrier, tomorrow will always bring still more worries. Being anxious is natural, but one of the keys to enjoying life is learning how to handle these worries. People learn to put their worries in proper perspective by acting, trusting, or putting them aside as is most appropriate for each one.

So, if these reactions are symptoms of normal anxiety or anxiousness, when does anxiety become a disease? How can you recognize when you have crossed the line from anxiousness to having an anxiety disease?

The physiological changes that occur when we are anxious can prepare us for better performance during a crisis—for flight or fight. Our senses are keen, our muscles are tensed, and our cardiovascular system is ready for increased exertion. The driver of the car may need to take quick evasive action. So might the couple in bed. The wronged wife may decide to use her black-belt training.

To a point these changes are normal and helpful, but beyond that point they are disruptive. Stage fright, or performance anxiety, is an example of acute anxiety. Many of us are nervous when we perform in front of a group. Speakers usually need to use the bathroom just before they go on stage. Mouths are dry, hands fumble notes, and knees shake. These symptoms are so common and so universal, that we have lecterns to hold up the glass of water, the notes, and the speaker. And, to a point, these symptoms do improve our performance. We are keener, more alert, and more inclined to do our best.

There is thus a peak level of anxiousness or alertness. Beyond that peak the symptoms start to get in the way. A speaker who has passed that peak may be so obviously nervous that the audience is distracted. A speaker beyond that peak may drop the notes in spite of the lectern, or need to clutch at the lectern just to stand straight.

The simple graph of Figure 1 illustrates this concept. The vertical arm of the graph, on the left, depicts increasing efficiency of performance. The horizontal arm shows increasing levels of alertness, or anxiety. You can see that performance improves as the level of alertness increases, but just to a maximum point. Beyond this peak, if anxiousness continues to increase, there is a rapid decline in performance. This leads quickly from peak performance to confusion or disorganization.

So how can you tell when anxiety is not normal? When anxiety symptoms interfere with your ability to function, and when they disrupt your life, they are not part of normal anxiety.

This seems like a relatively simple distinction, and it is for the

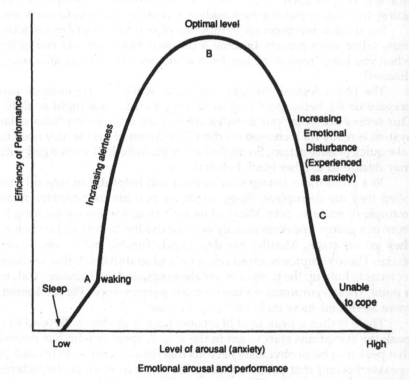

Figure 1. *Emotional Arousal and Performance. (From J. B. Cobb,* Postgraduate Medical Journal, *1982. Used with permission.)*[1]

person with sudden stage fright. If that person is too anxious to perform effectively, she or he needs to avoid performing or get some help. In the progression of most anxiety diseases, however, symptoms develop over a period of time and may at the outset be difficult to distinguish from other illnesses. For example, what if you have symptoms like tightness in the chest, shortness of breath, or night sweats?

The basic question to ask yourself is, "Are my symptoms the result of anxiety or something else?" Unfortunately, all of the symptoms describing anxiety can also be caused by a variety of other physical diseases.

HOW DO I KNOW

If you recognize that you are anxious, you need to ask yourself, "Are my symptoms out of proportion to this crisis?" Herein lies one of the great difficulties in early diagnosis. Most of us can't readily recognize, or even admit to ourselves, that our symptoms are disproportionate. "This crisis I'm in is enormous. It must be or I wouldn't feel so bad." "Anybody else in their right mind would be as upset as I am."

Answering the question, "Is my reaction out of proportion?" is not so simple. The answer depends partly on your own individual make-up. It also depends on the particular circumstances and the values you place on whatever is being threatened. For example, a farmer, after six weeks of no rain, watches his crops shrivel. An apartment dweller, facing the same drought, may lose the geraniums on the balcony. The natural occurrence, meaning the drought, is the same for both people, but the effects on their lives are vastly different. They are likely to respond differently as well. On the highway, after the near tragedy, one driver may shrug off the episode and resume his conversation. Another, after the same sort of episode, may need to stop by the side of the road and spend some time "getting himself together."

All of us have trouble looking at ourselves objectively. Sharing feelings with a family member or a trusted friend, someone who knows you and has spent time with you in other circumstances, may be the very best help. Your pastor or rabbi may be able to serve this role as well. You need to determine if you are having persistent symptoms, and whether these are due to normal anxiety, anxiety disease, or to some other disorder. If there is any doubt, your next step should be at least a phone call to your family doctor.

HOW THE ANXIETY DISEASE BEGINS

One of the ways our bodies apparently handle the effects of anxiety is chemically. In the course of looking for the cause of anxiety disease, scientists have made a fascinating discovery. They found that there are many chemical receptors in our brains. Each of these receptors is designed to accommodate a specific chemical compound. One of the most interesting discoveries is that one series of receptors seems to be designed specifically to accept a group of drugs we know as the benzodiazepines. The benzodiazepines are a family of drugs, all closely related to each other, which have antianxiety effects, or are "anxiolytic." This group includes Valium, Librium, and Xanax, among others. It seems highly unlikely that the Creator would have provided us with a set of receptors for a series of man-made drugs. It is much more likely that the body produces its own anxiolytic, a benzodiazepine-like drug. Intensive investigations are underway currently to identify and isolate such a drug.

Having identified this curious chemical receptor in people, scientists have looked for similar structures in other animals to provide models for study. Surprisingly, these same receptors were found in every species studied from humans down to the level of the shark, but not below that level. This would seem to indicate that all of us, including the shark, but not the fishes ranking lower than this on the evolutionary scale, are subject to the symptoms of anxiety. (Somehow it does not reassure me to think that if I were being chased by a shark, the shark might be just as nervous as I.)

Most of the examples I've presented so far are of people who have experienced anxiety symptoms in response to some crisis. These symptoms, in the face of a continuing crisis, may progress to become a disruptive anxiety illness. This is one of the ways that anxiety disease begins—as a persistent and disproportionate response to a bad situation.

Some of Paul's episodes of illness, in retrospect, did seem to be triggered by stressful events in his life. Had the symptoms occurred at the same time as the event, Paul (and his doctor) might have recognized them as evidence of anxiety. Sometimes this does occur, but often it does not.

A second way that anxiety disease often begins is "out of the blue." People who are not having a crisis in their lives, and are not experiencing any unusual stress or other precipitating factor, suddenly begin to have symptoms. They may be paddling serenely through life when they are suddenly assaulted by feelings of anxiousness, nervousness, or other physical symptoms for which there is no apparent cause, or no one to blame. This is what happened to Ruth. Life was lovely until she began to have these strange attacks of fearful symptoms. Something clearly went wrong with her body chemistry and she had no explanation, either psychological or physical.

Unfortunately, many people do not recognize that they are ill. They assume that somehow they are at fault and just need to "straighten themselves out."

A third, and very common way that anxiety disease starts is as an accompaniment to other ailments. One example would be a man who is having a heart attack and may be scared that he is going to die. This fright may be entirely rational, as indeed he could die during the attack. The anxiety itself may cause dangerous physiological changes; rapid heart beat, constricted circulation to the inner organs, and rapid breathing. All are likely to worsen his physical condition. This is not abnormal anxiety. Any of us might feel the same degree of anxiousness under similar circumstances. Since anxiousness becomes an anxiety disease when it interferes with how we function, this man is certainly suffering from a stage of anxiety disease.

As in some other illnesses, the body's response, instead of correcting a problem, makes the situation worse. For example, in hypertension the arteries are constricted. This results in a reduced blood flow through the kidneys. The same thing happens if we are bleeding profusely—less blood flows through the kidneys. The body's response is the same for either event—it produces chemicals that cause the arteries to constrict even further. This system works wonderfully if we are bleeding; it stops or reduces the blood loss. However, if the cause is high blood pressure, the constriction raises the pressure further and begins a vicious cycle.

The man with the heart attack may be harmed by his own body's response—a natural response, but considered a disease because it harms him. Prompt treatment of his anxiety with medication and appropriate reassurance may save his life.

However, many people, after the acute episode is past, and after leaving the intensive care unit and being assured that the immediate dangers are over, continue to feel symptoms of anxiety. This too may be another form of anxiety disease.

Almost any disease or injury is accompanied by anxiety and can be accompanied by anxiety disease. This is especially true in the case of ailments that are life threatening, or that the victim perceives to be life threatening. It is also true that any disease or injury can be followed by anxiety disease.

For reasons which no one fully understands, the complication of anxiety disease occurs more often with heart diseases than with any other group of ailments. A psychological factor may be the cause of this finding. We all know that we have only one heart, so we become fearful when it is not working perfectly. We know we have a spare eye, ear, lung, kidney, and yards of extra bowel, so we don't worry as much when they are in danger.

However, there could also be a structural or biochemical explanation. There is a common condition, just recently recognized, called mitral valve prolapse (MVP). This amounts to a sagging of part of the mitral valve, which is one of the main valves of the heart. It rarely causes any trouble and most people are unaware that they have it. However, several studies have shown that people with MVP are more likely than others to get an anxiety disease. If these studies are confirmed, it will be fascinating to find out if the connection is biochemical or psychological. It may help us understand the basic causes of anxiety disease.

The onset of an anxiety disease is not predictable. It can result from a prolonged or exaggerated response to stress; it can come entirely by itself; or it may show up as part of another disease. If it accompanies another disease it may be caused by the stress of that disease, occur spontaneously, or be caused by a combination of the two factors. To say that anxiety disease comes by itself or spontaneously, is just saying that the cause is not known and presumed to be due to some change in body chemistry. What causes those changes is still a big unknown.

SUMMARY

- Anxiousness is a normal part of being human.
- Anxiousness is useful to a point, but can become destructive.
- Anxiousness becomes anxiety disease when it interferes with normal functioning.

- You may need professional help to decide whether your symptoms are due to anxiousness, anxiety disease, or some other disease.
- Anxiety disease begins in three ways:
    As an exaggerated or prolonged response to stress.
    Spontaneously, with no precipitating stress.
    As an accompaniment to another disease.

Oh, the nerves, the nerves; the mysteries of
this machine called Man! Oh, the little that
unhinges it; the poor creatures that we are.
Charles Dickens

Chapter 4

Could It Be My Nerves?
The Meaning and Function of Symptoms

"It must be your nerves." The diagnosis of "nerves" has been around for centuries. It is a vague term usually used as an explanation for symptoms that don't seem to have any physical cause, such as anxiety and depression. But it is also used to describe normal anxiousness and other emotional reactions such as grief.

To many people the term "nerves" also has a pejorative meaning: your trouble is "just your nerves"—*mine is real*. When my patients use the expression "*just* my nerves" I usually answer, "Don't ever say *just* your nerves; they can cause some of the worst miseries you can get, and can be very hard to get rid of."

The term "nerves" is to the mind what "rheumatism" is to the muscles and bones. It's a useful kind of catch-all term, but one that doesn't describe anything very accurately. Anxiety diseases are *not* "just your nerves." They are a group of specific diseases separated from each other partly by differing causes, but mostly by the kinds of symptoms they produce.

Anxiety, as a clinical syndrome, is as old as recorded medical history. Hippocrates mentions it in his writings as far back as 400 B.C. In 1891 Dr. John C. Gunn, a general physician, described this syndrome

45

in his book *The New Family Physician* as an "indefinite condition of nervous irritability—a mixture of mental and physical disorders." He notes that the "mental emotions exert great influence over the body and its functions—the heart palpitates, the hands tremble, the face flushes, evidence of great nervousness or weakness." He speculates that this is more likely to occur in "those with sedentary habits or those who exhaust the brain by too great mental exertion." Recommended treatment was "exercise in the open air, cold showers, plasters on the spine, and a strengthening preparation of bitters."

One hundred years later one of the standard medical textbooks, *Cecil's Textbook of Medicine*, 16th Edition (W. B. Saunders Company, 1982) is not a great deal more specific: "Anxiety is an unpleasant mood of tension and apprehension . . . anxiety is a medical problem when it is excessive, inappropriate, or without obvious cause." There is no mention of the disease process, its biological causes, or the criteria for accurate diagnosis of the specific types of anxiety disease. This is the same information that was being taught to medical doctors as recently as 1982. It's not surprising that so much misunderstanding exists about these prevalent diseases.

Anxiety disease has been assigned many labels. My predecessor in practice used the term neurocirculatory asthenia to describe a patient with agoraphobia. Ruth, the patient we met earlier, was told by her endocrinologist that she had hyperdynamic beta-adrenergic circulatory state.

Diagnostic terms are used to describe a cluster of symptoms. Table 1 lists some of these diagnostic labels that have been used to describe anxiety disease. These terms have no specific definitions. They mean different things to different people, and are therefore useless. The variety of terms employed in the past, and unfortunately still employed to this day, reflects a widespread lack of understanding of how anxiety diseases are diagnosed, what causes them, and how they can be managed.

THE MEANING OF SYMPTOMS

Symptoms are part of the body's language—its means of communicating with us. Pain or discomfort, as when I touch a hot pan, means stop—I don't like this feeling. Otherwise, my hand might remain there until it is burned. Pleasing sensations like being hugged encourage

Table 1. *Former Diagnostic Labels
Used for Anxiety Disease*

Anxiety hysteria
Anxiety neurosis
Cardiac neurosis
Globus hystericus
Grand hysteria
Hysteria
Hysterical neurosis
Hyperdynamic beta-adrenergic state
Hyperventilation syndrome
Locomotor anxiety
Neurocirculatory asthenia
Soldier's heart
Vasomotor neurosis
Vasoregulatory asthenia

you to keep on doing something. It feels good. Both the pain and the pleasant sensation are part of the body's language.

As little children we begin to learn to pay attention to the language of our bodies. Late one night, when my daughters were very young, one came running to wake me complaining, "Daddy! I have oil! I have oil!" I awakened with dreams of a gusher until I realized she was reporting a symptom. She knew what indigestion felt like, even though she used the wrong term to describe it. (She had also learned the first step in treatment—waking Daddy—if you can.)

The body merely reports feelings. It doesn't process them or interpret them, and we are easily misled. I feel good about eating Hershey almond bars and could relish a whole pound. But usually I don't do it because I don't want to feel sick, get fat, or raise my cholesterol level. One of the markers of growing up is demonstrating the ability to interpret our feelings and act responsibly.

These are simple examples of feelings we have all learned to interpret, but there are others that are much more complicated or obscure, which we may not understand. A pain in the pit of the stomach feels like indigestion and most often is. However, acute appendicitis usually begins in the same way, even though the appendix is located in the lower right side of the abdomen. Pain in the left arm may be due to heart disease. Pain at the top of the right shoulder can be due to gallbladder disease.

In all of these instances the body is trying to tell us something. Unfortunately, it may require an interpreter to understand the signals. A health care professional, or interpreter, is not needed for an understanding of every feeling or symptom we perceive, but only those that persist, worsen, or that indicate one of the many danger signals we've come to recognize. They should also be called in when we experience symptoms that are just plain bewildering, such as cold sweats when it isn't cold, terror when there's nothing to be afraid of, or extreme discomfort for no apparent reason when leaving your house.

CAUSES OF ANXIETY SYMPTOMS

Anxiety, like other diseases, causes symptoms indicating that the body doesn't like what's going on. This chapter discusses the kinds of symptoms that anxiety disease causes, how these symptoms affect our bodies, and some problems involved in the diagnosis of these symptoms.

One of the unique features of anxiety disease is the enormous variety of symptoms it causes, affecting so many different parts of the body. To complicate matters further, the symptom patterns tend to keep changing. Adding to the problems in diagnosis is the fact that the symptom patterns often closely resemble the symptom patterns of other diseases. These features of anxiety disease often lead both the patient and doctor to a wrong impression or diagnosis.

When people get lobar pneumonia, it usually begins with fever, cough, and chest pain. By the next day they usually have higher fever and chills, pain while coughing, and shortness of breath. The next day, if not treated, all of the symptoms become worse and the patient also begins to cough up blood. The symptoms in this instance are dependable though severe; everyone who gets this disease always gets these same symptoms. The symptoms also make sense. The pneumococcus germs get into the lung and multiply. The poisons they send out cause the lung tissue to become inflamed, and the body responds with fever and chills. It is all very logical. This group of symptoms, in this pattern, almost always means pneumonia; the pattern doesn't look or act like nearly any other disease, with a few exceptions.

This is not the case with anxiety disease. Hardly any other disease at all is able to produce such an enormous variety of physical and mental symptoms. To add to the confusion, the symptoms vary from person to person and often vary in the same person from time to time. Our patient, Robert, first described his episodes of chest pain and the apprehension he felt about them. During the course of his illness he also had repeated episodes of abdominal pain, diarrhea, several attacks of severe dizziness, and many periods of depression.

When a patient describes a new set of symptoms before doctors figure out the old set, it can be very frustrating. Being human, we sometimes tend to blame the patient when there is an unexpected turn of events. "You didn't follow my instructions." Or some doctors may say, "It must be your nerves," or "It's all in your head." But anxiety symptoms are just as real as any other symptoms, and may be just as dangerous.

Edith is a middle-aged woman from another city who consulted me as a friend. She recited a long history of symptoms with which she had been suffering, off and on, for about two years. I obtained all of her medical records, at her request, and tried to review the entire story. I was appalled to find that during this time she had seen sixteen physicians. While her symptoms had changed considerably during this time, she really didn't feel any better than before she had embarked on this medical procession.

It has long been customary for physicians to consider "doctor shopping" as a sign of a personality problem or an emotional illness. This opinion may be totally backward. Doctors often become frustrated with patients who have anxiety disease, if they don't recognize it, and convey these feelings to the patient—by innuendo, by referral, or by outright rejection. "Doctor shopping" may sometimes be the sign of wise patients who recognize that they have a disease that each successive physician has failed to address.

Edith was such a person. She had an inadequately treated anxiety disease and was being referred from specialist to specialist as each new symptom developed, to search for diseases that weren't there.

To make matters even worse, she was treated with antibiotics for an unproven infection. She then had a reaction to the antibiotics and experienced a whole new set of symptoms, more referrals, and more tests.

Happily, once her anxiety disease was recognized she was able to get it under control.

In spite of the variety of symptoms and their tendency to change, there are specific qualities and patterns to the symptoms that now allow a diagnosis to be made with reasonable certainty, either by the patient or health care provider. There is a logic to anxiety symptoms, reasons why they occur and why they change. The logic, however, may not always be so obvious to either the patient or physician at first.

SELF-DIAGNOSIS

In several types of anxiety disease it is possible for people to make their own diagnosis. For example, a disabling fear of a danger that isn't real is a phobia. A continuing irresistible urge to wash one's hands many times per hour is an obsessive–compulsive disorder.

A young man named Elwood had been under my care for more than ten years before he told me that he had a phobia. He worked locally in an office on a full-time basis, but also had a part-time job as a basketball referee.

I thought I knew the family well, through home calls and after having delivered and helped raise their four children. I was amazed to hear him tell me that he'd realized he had a phobia many years before. He was totally unable to force himself to go into a tunnel or even a highway underpass. His solution was to accept it, and he found a job that kept him close to home, although he sometimes had to turn down refereeing jobs because of the travel required.

Elwood had diagnosed the phobia himself and was resigned to it. He told me about it only because his children were wondering why they could never go on trips to the shore like other kids did.

Usually the diagnosis is not so clear, even if suspected, and it is necessary to get professional help to sort out which symptoms are due to anxiety disorder and which can be ascribed to some other ailment. Self-diagnosis can be dangerous. Chest pain is often due to anxiety disease; but can also be due to heart disease—or to both. Failing to recognize and treat the anxiety can prolong the suffering indefinitely; failure to recognize and treat the heart disease can be fatal. A few years ago the distinction was much less important, because treatment for heart disease was not very effective, nor was the treatment for anxiety disease. Now that we have highly effective treatment for both, an accurate diagnosis is essential.

PAINFUL REALITY

Everyone dealing with anxiety, whether as a patient, family, or health care provider, needs to understand that the symptoms that characterize an anxiety disease are real—as real as a nosebleed or a broken finger. The symptoms are not imaginary, not psychologically determined, not an emotional disturbance, not "all in the head," and not a deliberate embellishment of normal feelings. The rapid heartbeat can be measured by an electrocardiograph. The diarrhea can cause dehydration like any other diarrhea. For the person who gets night sweats like Paul, the soaking wet pajama tops can almost be wrung out. We all know the reality of pain. Doctors can't measure it and no one can see it. Only the person feeling it can describe it and to that person it is an absolute and unquestionable reality. If I tell my wife I have a headache I will get sympathy. She knows what it's like to have a headache. If I tell my doctor, I will also get an investigation of the cause and some prescription or advice for relief. But if I complain of a "sort of vague achiness" or a "kind of floating sensation," the response to my complaints may be quite different. My wife is likely to question my sanity and the doctor my sobriety.

When you tell us, as doctors, about a symptom you are having, it automatically triggers a mental process in our heads. A whole list of possible causes traipses through our minds, with three to five chosen as the most likely candidates.

For example, if you complain of a pain in the abdomen, I will think of food or drink indiscretions, a gastrointestinal virus, appendicitis, peptic ulcer, gallbladder disease, pancreatitis, cancer of the stomach, etc. A few questions will narrow the field. Appendix out? Not appendicitis. Pain goes away with food? Possibly peptic ulcer. Pain is not severe? Not pancreatitis. No other symptoms at all? Probably not anxiety. Worse after certain foods like hot dogs, cabbage, chocolate? Likely gallbladder trouble. You point to where it hurts with the palm of your hand? Probably not peptic ulcer. You point to where it hurts with your finger tip? Probably peptic ulcer. The list keeps shortening with the answers.

Then a physical examination shortens the list even more. Tenderness under the right ribs means that it's probably gallbladder disease. Tenderness in the middle is more likely to be from peptic ulcer.

A few simple tests will help even further. Blood in the stool that is bright red, means a lower bowel problem. Dark blood is from the upper gastrointestinal tract. Blood that isn't visible but shows up on a chemical test could be from either location and could be due to any of the possibilities listed except gallbladder disease, appendicitis, gastroenteritis, or anxiety.

Then we may decide to do more specific tests such as x-rays, CAT scan, gastroscopy, etc. Or we may try a therapeutic trial of some regimen like avoiding certain foods, antacids, a liquid diet, etc. Or we may decide to do nothing and wait to see what happens. If it's viral it will clear up in one to two days. If it's appendicitis, the pain will probably move to the lower right quadrant of the abdomen within the next few hours.

All of this fits into a very neat decision-making process with the logic following a natural progression. It helps us as physicians to avoid the dangers of missing or delaying the diagnosis of some problem that could be easily fixed. But if you tell us about a symptom that is too vague to fit into one of our categories, or that we have never heard of before, or that you are not even sure of, we can get frustrated. You are telling us that our ten, fifteen, even twenty years of training and years of experience were all for naught.

Physicians respond to this dilemma in several ways. They may try to force the symptom into a known slot by saying, "what you really mean is. . . ," but of course, that isn't what you mean at all. Some physicians will become angry with you, describing you in the medical record as "a poor historian," as though you lacked the proper training for being sick, or for being a "good patient." A few others will respond with a quick "it's all in your head," or "it's just your nerves," either by their attitude or even in words. The more subtle will say that "perhaps it would be worthwhile to consider the possibility of seeing someone in a different field, maybe a nerve specialist."

Many physicians, like Edith's, begin a long series of studies, trying very hard not to miss an important diagnosis, and also to protect themselves from a possible malpractice suit. People sue more often for omitting tests than for doing too many, even though the tests may be expensive and carry some danger. If the real cause of the symptom is anxiety disease, the testing process may indeed be endless because there are no tests that prove the presence of anxiety disease. Furthermore, the symptoms of anxiety disease keep changing, and will constantly require new tests. Some patients crave the feeling that they have had "every test known to medical science." Fortunately, this is an impossible aspiration. New tests are always being devised and the old ones revised, faster than any one person could possibly use them.

It is my hope that your physician will consider the possibility of anxiety disease or depression as a possible cause. A few well-chosen questions may open up those possibilities. "What other symptoms do you have?" "How did it start?" "How do you sleep?" "What's going on in your life?" "How do you feel?" "Are you happy?"

These are good questions to ask if you're the doctor. But what can you do as a patient to help your physician? You could volunteer the answers to these unasked questions.

Several years ago a long-time patient came to see me because of shortness of breath and chest pain. I was alarmed and immediately launched into a routine of heart-related questions, and an examination of the cardiovascular system and a plan for some appropriate tests.

At that point my patient had the good sense and the insight to say, "Doc, could it be my nerves?" He stopped me in my tracks. I had not even considered the possibility of anxiety. I'm happy to report that he was right, and has since made a full recovery.

Never assume that your doctor, no matter how wonderful, knows more about you than you do. We only know what you choose to tell us or what we find out upon examination and testing. You don't have our medical knowledge, but it's your body and you know yourself much better than we ever can.

DESCRIBING THE SYMPTOMS

One of the other problems for people with anxiety disease is knowing what to tell the physician. Maybe they have never heard of a symptom like the one they are experiencing, or their symptoms keep changing, or it's just too hard to describe. This has often been the explanation my patients use when I ask them why they waited so long before coming to see me. Or sometimes they say, "I didn't want you to think it was all in my head," or worst of all, "I hated to bother you when there are so many people who are really sick."

Pain, bleeding, or a lump is simple—see a doctor. But tiredness, migrating pains, the inability to sleep, or just not feeling well—that's not so obvious.

Forty years ago I began my medical career as a solo practitioner in a small town of about 5,000 people in Hershey, Pennsylvania. One of my first patients was a woman named Henrietta who requested a home call. When I arrived at her home I was surprised to find that Henrietta seemed to be a very healthy looking fortyish woman who was dressed and seemed active. She explained to me that she hadn't been able to leave home for years because of her "condition." She was only able to get to the grocery store on the same block about once a week. When I pressed her about her "condition," she described a terrifying "all over moving feeling" that only happened when she left home.

Town folklore was that at one time Henrietta had been the most admired and beautiful woman in the village. She became betrothed to a man from out of town. On the day of the planned wedding he did not appear and hadn't been heard from again. Soon after this Henrietta withdrew from society and refused to leave the house, where she took care of her aged and ailing mother. Neighbors looked after both of them.

The family doctor, my predecessor, said it was her "nerves" and supplied her with "green medicine"—an elixir of the sedative pheno-barbital. She had steadfastly refused psychiatric consultation because she could not leave the house.

As a very new doctor I was amazed, perplexed, and frustrated by her continuously varying panorama of symptoms. Among the more prominent symptoms were joint pains and pains between the joints, diarrhea, constipation, stomach cramps, bladder problems, rashes I could never quite see, and a "trembling all over."

At first I thought my treatment was effective. Each group of symptoms responded to whatever I prescribed. But then I realized that they were always replaced by a new set. I had made no real progress and had no understanding of what was happening. The only thing that seemed to make life tolerable for Henrietta was the green medicine that I continued to supply. I was relieved to find that she never took more than the low doses I prescribed. I did try a kind of desensitization therapy, urging her to try to force herself to walk a few steps farther from the house each week.

Henrietta made some progress, but very slowly. Before she died, about 15 years later, of valvular heart disease, she actually made one trip to my office, which was three blocks away.

I have often wondered what kind of life Henrietta might have had if I had known as much about anxiety disease then as I do now; if we'd had present-day antianxiety drugs instead of only sedatives; and if we'd had the surgical skills to fix leaking heart valves or put in new ones. I learned to love Henrietta as much as my other patients and have always felt that she gave me more than I gave her. She gave me insight into anxiety disease that I would not have gotten in any other way.

UNDERSTANDING THE SYMPTOMS

One of the first and most important lessons I had to learn when I became a family doctor was to take every patient's symptoms seriously, no matter how bizarre, regardless of the fact that they were never mentioned in medical school or in the medical literature, and even if the symptoms didn't seem to follow anatomical patterns.

Oriental medicine views the body in its entirety, rather than in parts. Disease is considered to be a disordering or misarrangement of various life forces—a disruption of their normal flow patterns.

In western scientific medicine we study diseases according to their effects on various body systems. Most diseases attack, or represent a failure of a particular system, at least at the onset. This is the reason that so many of our specialties focus on one disease system, such as ophthalmology, cardiology, hematology, nephrology, neurology, etc. There is an -ology for every system and nearly every organ.

Based on anatomy and function, we usually divide the body into eleven systems:

1. Nervous system: brain, spinal cord and nerves, including the autonomic nervous system and sensory organs of sight, hearing, and smell
2. Integumentary: skin, hair, and nails
3. Respiratory: breathing apparatus from nose to lungs
4. Gastrointestinal: the food handling system, from mouth to rectum, including organs related to digestion, salivary glands, liver, gallbladder, and pancreas
5. Cardiovascular: heart, arteries, and veins
6. Musculoskeletal: bones, joints, muscles, cartilage and all connective tissue, tendons, and ligaments
7. Urinary: kidneys and bladder
8. Reproductive: sex organs
9. Endocrine: glands that produce hormones, especially the sex glands, thyroid, pituitary, and adrenals
10. Hematologic: blood, bone marrow, and spleen
11. Lymphatic: lymph nodes and tonsils

Since most diseases have their main effects on one system, the symptoms they produce are primarily located in that one system. For example, pneumonia primarily affects the lungs; high blood pressure damages the arteries and heart; cancer begins in one organ and affects that system first. Of course, there are some exceptions to this rule.

Anxiety disease is one of these. It is a direct cause of symptoms in at least nine of the eleven body systems. The only systems that seem to be exempt are the blood and lymph systems, which suffer no direct effects so far as we now know. There can, however, be indirect effects on these two systems. The person with anxiety disease may not be able to eat well and, as a result, will become anemic. There may also be direct effects that we do not yet understand. Several studies have shown that children in families who are under severe stress are more likely to have strep throat than other children. Perhaps stress, or anxiousness, may damage the immune mechanism.

Not only does anxiety cause symptoms in several systems at the same time, but the clusters of symptoms often change from time to time. On one of my home visits, Henrietta would complain of indigestion, diarrhea, and the inability to eat certain foods. On the next visit these symptoms might be gone and she would be intensely bothered by migrating pains in and between her joints. Another time it would be that "moving all over" feeling and a generalized trembling.

Even though there are an enormous number and variety of symptoms produced by anxiety disease and a tendency for these to change often, it is quite possible to identify groups of symptoms and patterns that will allow your doctor to make the diagnosis of an anxiety disorder with reasonable certainty.

SUMMARY

- Anxiety disease has been recognized for thousands of years and known by many names.
- Symptoms are part of the body's language: we need to listen, and sometimes we need an interpreter.
- The symptoms of anxiety disease can affect almost any of the body systems and tend to vary from time to time and person to person.
- Self-diagnosis is possible in some forms of anxiety disease, but can be dangerous.

- The transience and variability of anxiety disease symptoms can lead doctors astray. A perceptive patient can help.
- In order to recognize and understand anxiety disease we need to know what symptoms may be due to anxiety, what causes them, what they feel like, and what other disease can cause the same symptoms.

God may forgive you your sins, but your
nervous system won't.
                              Alfred Korzyski, 1879–1950
              (Polish born U.S. scientist and philosopher)

Chapter 5

Boogums, Snorklewackers, and Tigers

All we are, all we think, feel, smell, taste, see, every move we make, and the fact that we move at all—the very existence of our bodies—depend on the nervous system. It is our body's control tower, and is responsible for the workings of the entire mechanism. It is who we are. Without it we might all be petunias. Without our highly developed brain, we might all be monkeys. Since we expect a lot from this system, we might assume that it is fairly complicated. It is.

THE APPARATUS

The brain is shaped like a big onion that fits into a funnel with a lid on it—the skull. The narrow end is tucked into the narrow part of the funnel and extends down to form the spinal cord.

There are twelve pair of nerves, the cranial nerves, which are hooked up directly to the brain. They escape through the skull in conveniently arranged little holes and operate our face, eyes, ears, nose, mouth, and parts of the neck.

There are an additional thirty-two pairs of nerves, one pair for each vertebra along the spinal cord. These make up the peripheral nervous system, which is under our direct control. If we were cars, the peripheral nervous system would operate the lights, doors, windows, steering wheel, and other gadgets that require a driver to control them. We need another system to operate the engine, carburetor, alternator, and all the other things that need to happen automatically while we are busy working the lights, doors, windows, and steering. This system is called the autonomic nervous system. It consists of two chains of ganglia, or nerve centers, running parallel to the spine with branches to every organ in the body, including the blood vessels.

These two systems communicate through connecting fibers, mostly for gathering information. The brain receives information, coordinates it, thinks, and sends out messages based on what is happening and what we decide to do. All of these nerves, the cranial, peripheral and autonomic, extend to every tissue of the body.

HOW IT WORKS

Since we are such wonderfully complicated mechanisms, it is fortunate that much of our apparatus is set on automatic. If I step on a hot coal, I immediately jump back and only afterward do I realize what happened. As I indicated earlier, if I had to wait until the hot sensation message was relayed to the spinal cord, and then to the brain, and the brain recognized that the message meant excessive heat in the foot, and decided to move my foot, sent the orders and then moved my foot, I would have a well charbroiled sole.

The same kind of instinctive reaction occurs when the eye or the ear perceives a tiger. In response to a danger signal the autonomic nervous system responds reflexively, automatically, to notify the various organs to get ready for "flight or fight." The adrenal glands react to this emergency by squirting adrenalin into the bloodstream. The adrenalin prepares the circulatory system to provide more oxygen for the muscles and to cut down on all nonessential activities.

This is a significant concept in understanding anxiety disease. The nervous system is not purely an electrical system as we used to think. It is a chemical–electrical system.

Sensation messages come in and orders are sent out over an electrical circuit—the nerves. At every connecting point, or synapse, the flow of the electrical impulses is altered by chemical intermediaries called neurotransmitters. Each of these chemicals has a specific property that affects electrical impulses. Some chemicals block the impulses; others slow down the impulses. Still others speed up the transmission of the electrical flow across the gap from the end of one nerve cell to the beginning of another. Many of these substances are manufactured by specialized cells located at each synapse. The impulses are also influenced by adrenalin and other circulating chemicals.

SABRE-TOOTHED TIGER AHEAD

In this instance, the body speeds up the process of getting ready for action. What if, instead of a tiger, the ominous shadow turned out to be only the neighborhood sloth out for a stroll? The body's preparation would still be the same. The sensation that we felt would also be the same—a sense of apprehension or fear, pounding heart, fast breathing, sweating, and perhaps trembling. All of this would begin to ease off as soon as we were sure that there was no danger and no need to do anything.

Suppose we just imagined a tiger and there were no suspicious sights or sounds, and no tiger figure except in our own imagination? Perhaps Granny had been telling tiger stories around the fire at the cave, or we had dreamed of unfriendly tigers, or we just had an overactive imagination. Again, the response would be the same, the physical sensation would be similar and would continue until we were assured that the danger wasn't real. If we had a lively imagination, or a Granny who was an especially good story teller, our physical changes and sensations might continue for a long time. This is one of the effects of being a chronic worrier. The sensations, or symptoms of anxiety, go on and on. There is a continuing need to check for tigers.

ANXIETIES

Binkley is a small boy in the comic strip "Bloom County" who keeps all of his anxieties locked in a closet. He has seen them so often that he knows them all by name—Boogums, Giant Purple Snorklewackers, and others too hard to mention. His problem is that they have a tendency to get loose, or he can't resist peeking into his closet every now and then.

Whenever he does, the horrid looking monsters are there waiting to attack him (Figure 2).

Our problems are often the same. Even though we may know our fears and can call them by name, we have trouble locking them away and forgetting about them. It is not Binkley's fault that he has these anxieties. They are part of his life. It's not even his fault that he can't keep them safely locked away. They are part of him and something he has not yet learned to manage all of the time. Very few of us manage all parts of our lives as well as we would like.

Anxiety disease may be caused by an overresponse to any kind of danger signal. This was part of Paul's problem: fear of an early, forced retirement. Anxiety disease may also be caused by our response to imagined dangers.

But, there is a third, very frequent way, in which anxiety disease starts. Anxiety disease often happens to people without either a real or imagined danger. These people may be experiencing no stress at the time whatsoever. They have an abnormality affecting their neurotransmitters, the chemical–electrical system, which sets off and perpetuates the whole anxiety response.

The sensation of fear and the symptoms of anxiety are always extremely uncomfortable feelings, but they are lessened a bit if we know what frightened us, be it a tiger or a closet full of old ghosts. The sensation of fear when we *don't* know what is frightening us is far, far worse. How can we fight it, or run away from it, or even just put up with it, if we don't know what it is? This is the other way in which anxiety disease begins, and explains how people who feel entirely well, like Ruth, can be attacked by anxiety disease. Ruth was healthy, happy, enjoying her life, and free of any major stresses, when she had her first panic attack. What terror this must be to someone who has never experienced any similar symptoms, who is not ailing in any way, not feeling stressed, and who has never heard of panic disease. People who are chronically ill, who live with continuous stress, or who have had family members with anxiety symptoms, are at least aware that such things can happen to people.

ANXIETY CAUSES SYMPTOMS

Since the nervous system directly affects every part of the body, it's no surprise that anxiety symptoms also affect every part of the body. The list seems endless, and it is one of the reasons why people have

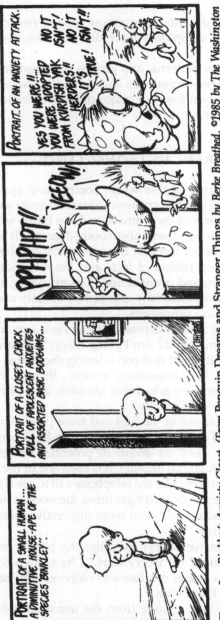

Figure 2. Binkley's Anxiety Closet. (From *Penguin Dreams and Stranger Things* by Berke Breathed. ©1985 by The Washington Post Company. By permission of Little, Brown and Company.)[2]

symptoms they can't describe, symptoms they've never heard of before, and sometimes symptoms their doctors have never heard of before.

However, there are patterns, and groups of symptoms, that many anxiety disease sufferers experience and some that we all experience. Since the nervous system has four major parts, let's look at the symptoms originating in each.

BRAIN AND SPINAL CORD

The organ in charge of this whole complicated apparatus is the brain, the intellect, the greatest creation so far (and so far as we know). It separates us from the rest of the animals, and, we hope, will separate us fast enough and far enough from sabre-toothed guests! It would be nice to think that this superior intellect of ours would be above all of this hubbub, this misinterpretation of facts and inappropriate responses, this pattern of reaction and overreaction. Unfortunately, the reverse is true. The mind is most profoundly affected by anxiety and produces a menagerie of disturbing symptoms.

The question that anxiety disease sufferers ask over and over again is, "Doc, am I losing my mind? Am I going crazy?" What worse feeling can there be than the thought that one is losing one's most precious and intimate possession? It is interesting to note, though, that I cannot remember ever having been asked that question by a patient who was actually losing touch with reality.

Excessive worry is one of the first and most persistent symptoms. Most of us worry to some extent. It seems to be a prerequisite for survival. It helps to keep us aware of potential dangers, to avoid physical, social, and financial disaster. It is even one of the ways that we show concern for each other like the telephone call to see if someone had a safe trip home. In sabre-toothed tiger times the worries may have been different but the reasons were even more imperative—safety, the next meal, or keeping warm.

But what is excessive worry? Even healthy people seem to differ, from "don't give a damn" to "worry wart." I have often noticed that in couples, when one partner is carefree and oblivious, the other seems to do the worrying for them both.

Excessive worry is a change from the usual attitude of concern toward life problems that is severe enough to interfere with your ability to function comfortably. It is worry that is out of all proportion to reality and to probability. It is worry about possibilities over which you have no control. "What if there's an earthquake?" "What if the pilot drops dead?" The "what ifs" march on in an endless procession of possible tragedy until the worry itself becomes the problem.

Robert was a great worrier. On the other hand, Elaine, his wife, seemed perfectly able to take each day as it came. She did not seem to worry, even about Robert, which was also a source of worry to him. "Why isn't she more concerned?" For each of his biweekly visits, Robert brought along a page, sometimes two, of worries.

- Pain on left side. Emergency Room. X-rays and blood tests. Said it was gas. White blood cell count low normal—what does this mean? Leukemia? Anemia? Low blood pressure?
- Dizzy spells.
- Elaine says sometimes I look grey around the eyes.
- Should I be taking so many pills—4½ per day?
- Slight stiffness in the back Wednesday morning. Never had it before.
- Thursday—bowel movement extra large, light brown, *no* odor. Why?
- Wednesday, forgot pill at noon. Anxiety attack after lunch. Getting worse?
- Dreamed we were at the seashore two times. Why?
- Felt nervous on way here.

Robert's appointments were rarely contained in the fifteen minutes allocated!

To the family member of a person with anxiety disease this excessive, apparently irrational worry is hard to understand. Admonitions such as "Let me do the worrying," or "It doesn't make any sense to worry about that," or simply "Don't worry," only aggravate the problem for the worrier, who then worries about how someone else can be so unconcerned.

To the excessive worrier advice such as "Don't worry, be happy" are not only useless, but quickly become nagging insults. Worry cannot be turned off like a faucet, obliterated by an act of will, or swapped for happy thoughts.

The worrier also has a tendency to "ruminate," an aptly descriptive word usually used to describe a cow chewing her cud. The worrier keeps bringing up old ideas, old worries, over and over and over, but with one important difference from the cow. This activity doesn't bring the worrier contentment. Old, seemingly forgotten worries, are brought up again and again and re-examined from every possible angle. Life, for the excessive worrier, seems to be a continuing struggle to swallow these cuds.

The nonworrier, or even the worrier when well, deals with recurrent thoughts rationally. Dangers are considered, as are their probabilities, and the possibilities of what could be done about it—move to a city where earthquakes are rare, cancel the trip, etc. Worry is put in its rational closet and left there.

Another activity of the brain that is disrupted in an anxiety-ridden person is sleep. Sleep patterns and the amount of sleep needed vary from person to person. Patterns also change as people get older. We know that this process is controlled by the brain, but how this works is still not well understood.

In anxiety disease, for whatever reasons, the normal patterns of sleep are disrupted. Most often the problem is manifested in difficulty falling asleep. In some people, sleep is repeatedly interrupted by anxious thoughts or disturbing dreams. The depressed person typically has no trouble falling asleep, but awakens much too early.

Insufficient sleep, or disrupted sleep, is often one of the reasons people with anxiety disease complain of overwhelming, unexpected fatigue. "But, Doc, I didn't do anything—I've often worked much harder than this and didn't get tired."

A third set of symptoms that originate in the brain is a feeling of irritability. This may show up merely as a touch of impatience or as a violent outburst of temper. It may also be as simple as an exaggerated startle response. Whereas the healthy person may react to an unexpected "Boo!" with a jump and a sloshing of the teacup, the person with anxiety disease is likely to drop the whole tray! This is not recommended as a diagnostic test. People with anxiety disease often describe themselves as feeling "on edge," "hyped up," "jumpy," or just "nervous." In Pennsylvania Dutch country we are likely to say we "feel all through-other" or "beside myself." This uncomfortable mood, if it continues for a long time, tends to alienate family and friends who otherwise could have been very supportive. This simply adds more troubles, or at the very least deprives the sick person of much needed support.

Another mood change that frequently complicates anxiety is depression. Studies have shown that seventy percent of people with anxiety disorders also have depressive symptoms at some time during the course of their illness. Like irritability, depression also causes profound and unexpected fatigue.

In anyone who is accustomed to being healthy, these symptoms, worries that won't stop, restless nights, and mood changes, will lead to introspection. "What is happening to me?" "Why can't I get hold of myself?" "There must be something really bad happening to me." Even previously fun-loving, carefree people can become totally absorbed in their own symptoms. A simple "How are you?" may trigger a whole recitation of bodily complaints. As troublesome as these "mental" symptoms are, both to the patient and to family and friends, they are really the lesser of the ways in which anxiety disease can affect the mind.

Severe anxiety interferes with basic thought processes. The anxious person often has great difficulty remembering simple recent events. This is extremely distressing, especially to those who are too young to make excuses for it because of their age.

Several years ago Melissa, the 42-year-old wife of an attorney friend, came to me for the first time. She was obviously deeply troubled. She had been a very healthy woman, highly educated, happy in her community and academic work, until the past few months. She still felt quite well physically, but had become increasingly forgetful. In the previous week she recounted several examples: she left one of her purchases at the store; she forgot her daughter's band practice; she forgot to return three library books. This, she said, was highly unusual for her. From this and some reading in her husband's medical–legal books she concluded that she had a frontal lobe brain tumor.

After a physical examination and CAT scan I was able to reassure her that there was no sign of any brain disease. When we explored further, however, it turned out that she was having anxiety symptoms, technically called "adjustment disorder with anxious mood," related to severe stress within the family. She was upset because her husband's law firm had disbanded. This meant that they would probably leave their community, find new positions, and enroll the children into a new school system.

I am happy to report that since their relocation she has felt entirely well.

It seems as though anxieties crowd out many of the thoughts and events of everyday living. This is very vexing to patients and frequently leads to misunderstandings within a family. One handy aspect is that this behavioral change can provide a clue to diagnosis. Anxious people often forget their appointments, or need to change them repeatedly, usually at the last minute, because of some forgotten conflict in schedule. A sensitive staff, instead of getting angry, will recognize that there is something unusual happening and will alert the doctor.

Patients with anxiety frequently call a few hours after their doctor's appointment to ask about details they have forgotten concerning their next appointment, medication, and other advice. This is especially true if doctors fail to put things in writing. Part of the same pattern of disruption is the loss of ability to concentrate. This can be very annoying in the course of daily living but extremely hazardous and totally crippling in the workplace. These problems present another reason why it is usually better to treat anxiety disease vigorously, instead of just letting it run its course.

Difficulty in remembering and an inability to concentrate fully combine to make the process of making even small decisions a great burden. "What should I wear?" "What should I do next?" "What kind of dressing do I want on my salad?"

Joan is a person who has been troubled with intermittent flare-ups of anxiety disease during the twenty years we have known each other. She and her husband are both now in their seventies. He works part-time for a fishing club, and one of his responsibilities is arranging fishing excursions.

Joan has always loved to fish and enjoys the camaraderie of the small groups. However, one of her first symptoms when she has a recurrence of her anxiety disease is difficulty in making decisions. She simply cannot decide which clothes to take for the trip. As she described it, she lays out on the bed all of the clothes she could possibly want—but she simply cannot make the final decision of what to put in the suitcase. At one point, this became such an overwhelming concern that she simply stopped going on all overnight trips.

When a person has difficulty making small decisions, it is extremely hazardous to make big decisions about relationships, commitments, jobs, health care, and financial choices. The intense anxiety of being pushed to make a decision may force people to make precipitate choices just to relieve the pressure of the anxiety.

This aspect of anxiety disease—disruption of normal decision-making processes—is one of the most disturbing, and even frightening, consequences of untreated anxiety. I believe that the unfortunate outcomes of poor choices due to anxiety disease may be far more widespread than we know, or than we even know how to measure.

Cranial Nerves

Blinking is an example of a nervous response to anxiety affecting a single muscle group. Blinking is necessary; it helps keep the eyeball bathed in fluid like a windshield wiper in reverse. The average number of blinks per minute is about 14. People who study human behavior count the blinks of people under duress, as an index to their degree of anxiousness. This can be an interesting exercise with TV talk shows. Count the blinks per minute of the interviewer and the interviewee to see which one is more nervous.

One of my patients, an active businesswoman, had a marginal blepharitis, which is an inflammation of the margin of the eyelids. This causes some redness and swelling, annoying itching, and frequent blinking. Treatment consists of warm wet compresses and various medicated creams. These treatments usually control, but do not cure, the ailment. This patient's unrecognized anxiety disease greatly magnified the problem for her. She sought help from numerous specialists in two academic medical centers. It was not until I finally recognized and helped her control her anxiety disease, that she found relief. In this instance the anxiety disease did not cause the inflammation of the eyelids, but it did focus her whole attention on that spot and made her symptoms ten times worse.

The squinting of one eye is also a frequent symptom of anxiety disease. Treatment doesn't help much unless the underlying cause is found. The cause can be anxiety, but it can also be many other diseases. Some of these causes are benign, like a viral infection, and some are dangerous, like a tumor.

Since the cranial nerves involve the face and neck, many other symptoms are possible such as twitching or spasm of other facial muscles. Tension or spasm of the jaw muscles result in chattering teeth. People who have this kind of muscle tension sometimes grind their teeth while asleep. If untreated this can cause severe dental problems.

Another frequent symptom is a sensation of a lump in the throat, the feeling we get at some poignant moment as when the folded flag was handed to John F. Kennedy's widow. With anxiety disease, however, this lump persists and becomes quite frightening. It feels as though we are swallowing over a hill, and as though it might strangle us if it got any larger. This symptom is caused by spasm of the muscles in the throat. It is reassuring to know that it is not possible for this "knot" to become so big as to prevent breathing or swallowing. That knowledge helps allay some fear, but it doesn't make the lump go away. This is true for most symptoms of anxiety disease. It helps to know what's happening, but it doesn't remove the symptoms or cure the disease.

Both anxiety and anxiety disease also frequently affect our speech, both the voice itself and our manner of speaking. Many of us have been bothered by a quavering voice while speaking in public or sometimes even by a total voice failure. We try to say something and no sound comes out. Though very embarrassing, it is very human. Our manner of speaking may also be affected from sputtering and stuttering to the inability to find the right words. Or we may talk too softly, too loudly, or too fast. All of these symptoms are just part of the everyday anxiety of life.

In anxiety disease, though, the symptoms persist even when there is no obvious reason to be upset. I have had a patient, Agatha, whose anxiety disease has been intermittent for more than thirty years. Her most noticeable symptom, not the one that bothers her most, but the one that bothers me most, is her speech. Normally her speech is soft, rapid, organized, and intelligent, and her visits to me are infrequent. When she has a flare-up of anxiety disease, the staff all recognize it before she arrives. Deciding on an appointment time takes several phone calls, with one or two changes and then she may arrive at the wrong time.

When I see Agatha she will be sitting in the examining room furiously writing lists of symptoms, thoughts, and events she wants to tell me about. If I am five minutes late the list may grow to forty or more items. As soon as I enter the room she is likely to say,

> This back pain is killing me doctor and Jack thinks I take too many pills anyway why is it always on my left side the whole left side is no good my sister is much worse the one in the nursing home but sometimes it's on the right side do you think it's my nerves again Jack wants me to go along on a trip but you said I don't have to I guess it is anxiety again but why don't the pills help maybe I should start taking them again . . .

When I finally stop her, often with a gentle hand on her shoulder, she is able to laugh a little, recognize what is happening, and agree to begin "the pills" again and to come back regularly. But when I take my hand off her shoulder, it is like turning on the shower again. It is no wonder that one of her most dreaded symptoms is physical exhaustion.

None of these responses seem well designed to help us face or run from danger. Chattering teeth may sound to us like a machine gun, but to our prehistoric predator, it probably just sounded like dinner.

Peripheral Nervous System

A generalized response of the peripheral nerves can cause shaking or trembling all over the body. People often describe a sensation of "being weak in the knees." This happens when muscles quiver instead of locking the knees in place so we can stand unassisted. I, personally, never speak in public unless I have a lectern or pulpit. I say I need something sturdy to "hold my notes," but it's really to hold me, just in case.

Some people, in response to a threat, are literally "paralyzed with fear" and are unable to take any useful action. Perhaps this is a kind of evolutionary aberration of the "play dead" response of some animals, such as the opossum. These little creatures move too slowly to escape predators, so when threatened they just "go limp" and are actually temporarily paralyzed. No self-respecting carnivore will then attack. Unfortunately, this response has proven to be very ineffective against the Jaguars, Mustangs, and Cougars of the interstate.

Another function of the peripheral nervous apparatus is to relay sensations. These include the feelings of pleasure, pain, and everything else in between. During anxiety, they, too, can become a problem.

One of the basic feelings we experience during anxiety is called, in the official description of anxiety disease, "vigilance and scanning." This means a heightened awareness, feeling on edge, nervous, worried, apprehensive, and endangered. As a result of this supersensitivity, we get false signals from our sensors or we may simply misinterpret normal signals. We might feel creepy, crawly sensations of the skin, or hot or cold sensations. The soft sounds of a cat on the stairs may seem like the stealthy tread of a burglar or its shadow like that of a tiger.

One day a state policeman friend called me with urgent concerns about my patient, Agatha. He was convinced she had completely lost her mind. At the time, Agatha was experiencing a flare-up of anxiety disease and had been to my office the day before. One of her more troublesome symptoms was "vigilance and scanning." She was expecting something calamitous to happen every minute. The state police officer, of course, was completely unaware of this. He was a neighbor of Agatha and Jack and merely stopped at the house to see if they had seen his missing cat. When Agatha opened the door and saw him, uniform and all, it seemed to confirm her worst fears, even though she didn't know what they were. She dissolved into total incoherence.

The startled officer knew that Agatha was one of my patients, and called me. I called Agatha at once and after a short while she began to put the pieces into perspective. Now she will even joke about it, but at the time it was an overwhelming terror.

Sometimes the usual sensations of body functions or of moving muscles and joints may actually become painful. This does not mean that the organs, muscles, or joints are diseased although they may feel that way. Nor are the feelings imagined or "dreamed up." The brain is either receiving the wrong data or is misinterpreting the data it receives. Either way, the feelings are the same. These feelings, unexpected and unaccountable, add more fuel for the imagination and the level of anxiety spirals upward.

Autonomic Nervous System

In response to danger signals, the autonomic system really does prepare us either to fight or flee. The whole circulatory system is altered and other systems are virtually shut down. This is a marvelous arrangement, but also poses new problems. What happens if we don't want to fight or flee? What if we can't identify the danger we need to face or avoid? What kind of sensations does all of this internal rearranging cause? If we can't control it, and don't want it, what happens next? The answers to these, and similar questions, depend on the particular system or organs affected, so each of these will be discussed separately.

SUMMARY

- All parts of the nervous system, brain and spinal cord, cranial and peripheral nerves, and autonomic nervous system, have key roles in anxiety symptoms.
- The flow of electrical impulses in the nervous system is affected by chemical intermediaries, called neurotransmitters.
- Any threat, real or imagined, may set off the anxiety response.
- Anxiety disease can occur as an overresponse to danger, or an overresponse to an imagined danger.
- Anxiety disease also happens to people with no real or imagined danger, and no stress whatsoever.
- Frequent symptoms of anxiety disease involving the brain are excessive worry, disturbed sleep, irritability, depression, and difficulty in thinking.
- Some of the cranial nerve symptoms are frequent blinking, twitching of the face, teeth grinding, lump in the throat, and disruption of speech.

- Symptoms of anxiety in the peripheral nervous system include trembling, unusual skin sensations, and painful muscles and joints.
- The autonomic nervous system prepares the body for flight or fight by "revving up" the cardiovascular apparatus and shutting down other systems.

I hav finally kum to the konklusion that a
good reliable sett ov bowels iz wurth more tu
a man, than enny quantity ov brains.
            Henry Wheeler Shan, 1818–1885
(Josh Billings)

Chapter 6

When the Body Speaks
Symptoms of the Skin, Respiratory, and Gastrointestinal Systems

The patterns of symptoms and their progression, along with the sequence and circumstances in which they develop, constitute the history of a particular illness. This history, plus the findings of a physical examination, provide all of the information usually needed to make an accurate diagnosis of one of the different types of anxiety disease.

Most organs respond in a programmed way to the chemicals set off by a threat or an anxiety-producing situation. Anxiety can also be produced by an imaginary problem, as the old Scottish prayer says, by "ghoulies and ghosties, long leggety beasties and things that go bump in the night." The body's reactions to imaginary dangers are the same as to real dangers. It is not the body's job to know the difference between them. To an extent, we do have some control over our imaginary ills, or at least we can learn to exert some degree of control of our reactions to them.

Anxiety symptoms are often *not* due to a real danger or to an imagined danger or even to the presence of another disease. Much more importantly, *anxiety symptoms are often caused by the release of certain body*

chemicals without the impetus of any real or imagined stress in otherwis
healthy people. You don't have to be sick or upset or stressed in any way
to get an anxiety disease. Ruth was a happy, healthy, robust, well
adjusted, mature woman when she suddenly began to have pani
attacks. They were not a response to stress, nor did she imagine them

It is not necessary to know the cause of an anxiety disease in orde
to understand the symptoms. Each of the body's systems has its own
way of responding to anxiety disease. One practical way to study this i
to review one system at a time, but it is important to remember that in
the body all of these symptoms are related to each other and many may
be happening at the same time. The response of one system may cause
symptoms in another. For example, Robert's chest pain may have triggered more rapid breathing, causing hyperventilation, which caused
the numbness and tingling in his hands and feet.

In considering each system I will review its normal functions, how
it responds to anxiety, the symptoms and disruptions that anxiety may
cause, and how this reaction affects other systems. I also will show how
all of these same symptoms can be caused by other diseases.

THE SKIN

The purpose of the skin is to keep us all tidily wrapped, warm, and
protected from the environment, and I suppose, to make us a bit more
presentable. It is the largest organ of the body, nearly 20 square feet. It is
the principal means by which we sense and interact with our surround-
ings, allowing us to feel heat, cold, touch, pleasure, and pain. It is so
sensitive that we can feel an ant walking on us and know exactly where
it is. We can learn to read by feeling the little bumps that are used in
Braille.

Through perspiration and subsequent evaporation, the skin helps
control our internal temperature. Our blood vessels can constrict to
conserve heat or dilate to aid in cooling.

The skin reacts in its own peculiar way to signals of anxiety. Often
the blood vessels under the skin constrict, causing a cold sensation.
Also, the sweat glands may become overexcited, resulting in cold
sweats. This can take place all over the body, but most often, occurs in a
local area such as the small of the back, the soles of the feet or the palms.
Cold, sweaty palms are one of the things a doctor looks for when
shaking hands with a patient.

Sometimes the blood vessels of the skin dilate and the skin becomes flushed. This also usually occurs in a particular area: the face, neck, and upper chest, during a period of anxiety or embarrassment. Additionally, the little hairs of the arms, back of the neck, and upper back often raise, causing us to feel "goose flesh" or a prickly sensation. This may represent a reflection of our ancestry. Many animals, most notably cats and porcupines, are able to raise their hair at a time of danger. This makes them look much more formidable to an attacker. We seem to have lost something in evolution; our present-day "goose bumps" hardly seem effective for frightening off a charging tiger.

Another annoying and quite common skin symptom is paresthesia. This is a peculiar skin sensation of something creeping or crawling, or feelings of hot and cold, burning, itching, or even a sense of tightness of the skin. These feelings can be very discomforting and puzzling to a victim, especially in view of the normal appearance of the skin. They cause no visible damage, although they may be accompanied by flushing or goose flesh. It is disturbing to find bugs crawling on the skin; but to feel the crawling and find no bugs is even more disturbing! This is the sort of symptom that makes people wonder about their own sanity.

Other common skin changes are hives or neurodermatitis. Hives are welt-like lesions, sometimes large, which come and go and may itch intensely. Neurodermatitis is a fine itchy rash, which when first seen by a physician is often already scratched open because of the intensity of the itching. Hives and rashes can sometimes be traced directly to stress.

I had a friend in medical school who was an excellent student, a calm and self-confident person. He studied hard and was always well prepared for class. However, when we had major examinations, his skin always responded—he got red, itchy spots on the palms of both hands. These began about a day before the exam and continued for a day or two afterward, then gradually faded. Fortunately, it didn't interfere with his test taking. It did make him the brunt of much joking though, especially since similar spots can occur with syphilis.

When I was new in practice, and our family was quite young but teeming, we had a housekeeper who had become so endeared to all of us that we called her Mom. When she needed some major surgery I agreed to scrub in as an assistant to the surgeon. There were many complicating factors, and I worried about the outcome. On the day of surgery, I developed such huge hives on my hands that I was unable to scrub and had to find another doctor to serve as surgical assistant. My

Table 2. *Skin Symptoms and Some Causes Other than Anxiety*

Symptoms	Other Causes
Excessive sweating	Heat, exercise, chronic infections
Flushing	Heat, heat flashes, fever, emphysema
Paresthesia	Neurological diseases (e.g., multiple sclerosis)
Hives	Allergy to something taken internally (food or drugs)
Rash	Skin allergy
Itching	Allergy, scabies, jaundice

body had responded to the stress by preventing me from continuing that stressful situation. The surgery went well, and there were no complications for the patient or me; my hives disappeared as rapidly as Mom improved.

Anxiety can be the cause of any of these skin symptoms, and they could be signs of anxiety disease (see Table 2). The symptoms can also be due to a variety of other causes. Determining which is which— anxiety, anxiety disease, or another cause—is dependent on the history of the present illness and the results of a physical examination.

THE RESPIRATORY SYSTEM

The respiratory system is the body's whole breathing apparatus. We take air in through the nose and mouth to the lungs where oxygen is extracted from it as needed and replaced with the carbon dioxide we need to get rid of. Along with that there is some loss of water, visible when you see your own breath on a cold day. The controls for this are all nicely handled by the autonomic nervous system. We don't have to think about how fast or how deep or when to breathe.

When confronted with danger we expect to use a lot more energy suddenly and therefore we will need a lot more oxygen. The system is then activated to make us breathe deeper and faster. This arrangement works very well as long as we are running or fighting or are physically active in some way, because we are using up more oxygen and expelling the appropriate amount of carbon dioxide.

The trouble comes when the danger is not real and we don't really need to exert ourselves. As we breathe deeper and faster, we continue to expel carbon dioxide—too much carbon dioxide. The first symptom of this loss is dizziness, as patients sometimes experience when a doctor says "take deep breaths." The dizziness, while uncomfortable, usually causes no serious trouble and soon disappears when the person resumes normal breathing. To many people this dizziness is frightening, especially if they don't know the cause. They quite naturally respond to this fear by breathing still deeper and faster. Further loss of carbon dioxide will cause numbness and tingling first, then cramping, and then spasms of the feet and hands. This pattern of breathing is called hyperventilation and is a common cause of some of the symptoms of anxiety disease. However, the vicious cycle can be broken by breathing in and out of a paper bag. This helps retain carbon dioxide, which in turn acts as a brake to slow the breathing process.

I once received an urgent request for an emergency home call for an unconscious teenage girl. When I arrived I found the entire family, plus a few neighbors, gathered around. My patient was lying on the floor breathing heavily. She had regained consciousness, but her eyes were dilated widely and she was breathing both fast and deep. She was beginning to have spasms in both hands, making her fingers clutch together uncontrollably.

It was easy to recognize that she was hyperventilating. I cleared the room and was soon able to talk her into relaxing and breathing slowly. She recovered quickly and then related how she had been having a verbal battle with her mother. Both she and her mother were very excitable people. "Curing" her immediate problem was easy. The counseling of both mother and daughter to try to prevent recurrences was much more difficult. Explaining to the parents, who both had a limited understanding of English, what had happened in a way that made sense, proved almost impossible.

Ordinarily we are quite unaware of our own breathing. An exception occurs during pregnancy. About the fourth month many women suddenly become aware of their own breathing, which makes them very uncomfortable. As the baby grows and the womb rises up out of the pelvis, it occupies much more abdominal space and there is less room for the diaphragm to contract. This forces the pregnant woman to breathe more with her chest muscles, which often is perceived as a shortness of breath. Most women soon adapt and again become unaware of their breathing.

In anxiety disease this smooth pattern of breathing is rudely interrupted. People often become keenly aware of the need to breathe, which may result in deep sighing. It also can lead to a series of changes caused by the loss of carbon dioxide. Carbon dioxide is supposed to serve as a governor for the breathing controls. Loss of this control causes breathing to become more and more rapid, lowering the carbon dioxide level even further. This lowered level triggers changes in the smaller muscles. The muscles of the hands and feet contract in claw-like spasms. If the loss of carbon dioxide continues, there will be contraction and spasms of the big muscles as well, eventually leading to convulsions.

The combination of increased breathing, along with the tendency for secretions to dry up—another autonomic nervous system effect—often leads to a dry cough. This is the kind of cough you often hear in an audience when a person is nervous. At one time, I was a member of a committee where the chairman had a kind of clearing-the-throat nervous cough. At times this would become very frequent and quite harsh. He was much annoyed by it, but unable to control it. As his family doctor I knew there was nothing wrong internally, and no disease of his breathing system. During our long, and sometimes intense, meetings, some of the other members (not me!) used to do a "cough index," counting the number of coughs per minute. This index served as a reliable nonverbal guide about how the chairman was feeling about each issue.

There is a good side to all of this breathing trouble. There are simple and inexpensive respiratory function tests that can be done quickly in a doctor's office that will help you find out whether your breathing trouble is due to emphysema, heart disease, anxiety, asthma, or anything else.

The catch is that the tests are most useful in showing anxiousness or part of an anxiety disease if they are done while you are having the symptoms. They measure the actual depth and effectiveness of your breathing. If your respiratory function has already returned to normal, the rapid breathing, spasms, and dryness quickly disappear. However, the tests are still useful because they can show evidence of the other respiratory diseases, even if symptoms are not immediately present.

As with the skin, respiratory symptoms can be due to anxiety, anxiety disease, or other causes (see Table 3). Unlike the dermatological symptoms, however, respiratory symptoms can be evidence of life-threatening disease. Professional help may be essential to determine the diagnosis.

Table 3. *Respiratory Symptoms and Some Causes Other than Anxiety*

Symptoms	Other Causes
Shortness of breath	Exertion, pregnancy, emphysema, heart failure
Fast, rapid breathing	Exertion, blood clot in the lung, collapsed lung
Dry cough	Respiratory infection, allergy, air pollution, lung tumor

THE GASTROINTESTINAL SYSTEM

This is the entire food processing system, from taste to waste. Most of the organs of this system are controlled by the autonomic nervous system, except at both ends, which are under voluntary control. The whole arrangement is responsive to real or perceived threats. In many of us the first and most prominent symptom of anxiousness occurs in this system. In fact, the gastrointestinal response is so much a part of human nature that we have all experienced it in some form, such as dry mouth, heartburn, aching in the pit of the stomach, cramps, or diarrhea.

In the era of roaming sabre-toothed tigers this represented a very useful reaction. The digestive process requires the use of a large part of the blood supply. Hence the old adages, "Don't exercise on a full stomach," and "Don't swim for twenty minutes after eating." When we are threatened, or even think we are threatened, the extra blood supply that had been so happily digesting our nuts and berries, is suddenly shut off. Instead, it is shunted directly to the muscles so that they are prepared to run or do battle. Most of the digestive juices from the salivary glands, pancreas, and liver are turned off. These arrangements work harmoniously for the purpose of immediate action, but there is a price: food cannot be fully digested without these juices. The result of semidigested food is indigestion, gas, belching, and bloating.

The adrenalin released in response to our glimpse of the sabre-toothed tiger has profound effects on the rest of the gastrointestinal system as well. The entire hollow plumbing system—esophagus, stomach, small and large bowel, gallbladder and rectum, including the sphincters that regulate the flow—is lined with muscle fibers controlled by the autonomic nervous system. Muscle fibers can only do two things: contract or relax. During digestion they contract rhythmically, propelling food along its way in an orderly fashion. They open and close sphincters in a timely and socially acceptable manner. However, when they respond to danger they only contract, causing the whole tubular system to constrict and the sphincters to shut tightly.

If we are not too distracted by the tiger, we may be bothered by many symptoms. Esophageal spasm is often felt as chest pain. Stomach and esophageal spasm also may cause vomiting. Spasm of the bowel may result in diarrhea, at times explosive as the tight sphincter suddenly lets go.

Under some circumstances there may be a benefit to these reactions. Emptying our gastrointestinal system at both ends helps prepare us to run, and may even cause our hungry tiger to reconsider. For many people the gastrointestinal system is the major target of anxiety symptoms. While some of these symptoms are part of our universal human experience when we feel anxious, in the person with anxiety disease these may be severe, chronic, disabling, dangerous, and even life threatening. The most frequent symptoms are dry mouth, heartburn, stomach distress, abdominal discomfort, and diarrhea.

Dryness of the mouth, or the inability to spit, is ordinarily just an annoyance, but it can be a useful reminder that you are anxious, even when you are not consciously aware of it. Severe dryness can make speaking very difficult. It's the reason for the glass of water on the speaker's lectern. This symptom is a good reminder that we are all subject to the discomforts of anxiety.

Difficulty in swallowing, or dysphagia, may be a symptom of anxiety or of anxiety disease, or it may be a symptom of many forms of disease of the esophagus. With esophageal disease the difficulty usually begins gradually, with problems in swallowing larger bites of food. Esophageal disease progresses slowly, rather than being intermittent as with anxiety or anxiety disease. There are two reassuring facts that every anxiety patient should know. First, this kind of lump-in-the-throat spasm does not lead to other diseases of the esophagus. And second, no matter how large the lump gets or how tight the throat feels, it is physiologically impossible for it to close the esophagus completely.

Heartburn is a burning pain in the mid-chest area, often described as a hot sensation. Sometimes it seems to rise up to the throat and can be accompanied by a brackish taste or even some regurgitation of stomach contents. Unlike true heart pain, heartburn always stays in the mid-chest area and doesn't radiate to the arms. It feels like it needs a good cold drink to "put the fire out," but this usually makes it worse. It can almost always be relieved with one or several doses of an antacid such as Maalox®, Camalox®, Tums®, Rolaids®, Gelusil®, Mylanta®, or even plain baking soda—not recommended for frequent use because of its high sodium content.

People who know they have anxiety disease may be able to avoid some symptoms by eating very light, easily digestible foods when they are under stress or know they are likely to become stressed. For example, they can include such foods as apple juice, and fresh fruits, but only if they are very ripe. Hot or cold cereals are tolerated well, especially with skim milk. Nonfatty soups and simple starches such as potatoes, rice and pasta are recommended. Some vegetables seem to be easily digested, especially the root vegetables—carrots, beets, and turnips. I suggest avoiding raw vegetables and those with tough outer coverings such as corn, and those with strong flavors like onions or rutabagas. Known gas-producing vegetables like cabbage or beans may be a problem. The most easily digested meats are fowl, especially the white meat, and fish. Simple desserts such as puddings, sherbet, and gelatin are easily digested, but those high in fat and sugar are best avoided. Anything fried or fatty or highly seasoned should be avoided. So should coffee and alcohol.

These precautions are useful for people who have gastrointestinal symptoms from their anxiety disease, but only if they have been able to discern some pattern and some predictability to their symptoms. Following a diet such as this without a clearcut reason would be adding an unnecessary hardship to a person who is already severely troubled.

Many of the stresses and strains of everyday life are predictable, and these are what lead to symptoms of anxiousness. Anxiety disease is different. It often has nothing to do with stress, although this can make the symptoms even worse. The occurrence of symptoms is quite unpredictable. Weekends are not likely to be any better than week days. Robert described this. He felt that his symptoms would pass after a long Thanksgiving weekend of relaxation. Instead, they got worse.

Peptic ulcer is a disease that often appears to be precipitated by a period of intense mental or emotional stress. Although it has been difficult to prove or disprove conclusively, I believe that severe anxiety disease is one of the causes of this disease.

Peptic ulcer disease, or duodenal ulcer, begins with an irritation of the lining of the duodenum, the first part of the small bowel. The disease is confined to the area just an inch or two past the stomach. If the process continues, an ulcer or hole develops in the lining at that location. If the ulcer erodes into a blood vessel there will be bleeding, which can be severe to life threatening. The ulcer also may erode through the entire wall of the duodenum causing a perforation. This usually results in sudden and extreme abdominal pain, a surgical emergency.

The stomach responds to anxiety by producing more hydrochloric acid, which is one of the digestive juices useful for handling food. If it is not absorbed by food in the stomach, or by antacids, this excess acid serves as an irritant. The result is "butterflies," "knots," or cramps, or just an uncomfortable sense of fullness.

One of the causes of peptic ulcer is an excess of hydrochloric acid in the stomach. Early symptoms of ulcer disease are vague fullness, discomfort, or aching in the pit of the stomach—in the middle, just south of the breastbone. It usually is relieved by eating food or drinking milk. Later, as the ulceration begins, the pain becomes more sharply localized. Patients will point to the spot with one finger, while before they would use their whole hand.

How can you tell if the hurt in the pit of your stomach is due to anxiety or the beginning of an ulcer? You can't, because physiological changes from anxiety disease might be contributing to the start of an ulcer. This is one of the most graphic reasons that anxiety disease should be treated promptly and thoroughly, rather than just being endured in hopes that it will go away.

Abdominal cramping, with or without diarrhea, is an especially troublesome symptom. It is variable, intermittent, and unpredictable. It usually does not seem to be related to particular foods. People often tend to identify symptoms with one particular food, but then find the same symptoms occur with a different food, or do not recur when the original food is tried again. Eliminating each suspected food soon leads to an extremely restricted and lopsided diet. I always urge a patient not to eliminate a food from the diet on a single suspicion, but to try it several more times in very cautious amounts.

Cramping can be a mere annoyance, recognizable by the person as related to other anxiety symptoms, or it can occur by itself and be very misleading.

Some years ago, on the Saturday before Easter, a young priest called me. He was having moderately severe, intermittent pain in his abdomen. He had no nausea, vomiting, diarrhea, or any other symptoms. He did remember having another attack like this just before he'd graduated from seminary. Now he was worried about appendicitis, not as a frightening disease, but as a threat to his Easter celebration, which was the high point of the year for him.

When I examined him I found his abdomen a little tender in the right lower area, but with no definite signs of active disease. His temperature and pulse were both normal. I did a blood count that was also normal.

Since Easter morning was less than 24 hours away, we decided to watch the situation closely and he agreed to stay on a clear liquid diet and get as much rest as he could manage. I examined him again on Easter eve. The pain had continued and yet the findings on examination were the same. I was encouraged because appendicitis usually progresses over a period of six to twelve hours.

Easter morning he assured me that although he had a little pain, he felt well otherwise and could easily manage the service. During the next few hours the pain disappeared.

We would never have understood the origin of this pain, except that it became a pattern, repeated several times during the years he was under my care. There were additional episodes, not again at Easter, but always connected with some major event in his life. When we both recognized this, he was able to avoid most of the symptoms by staying on a very light diet whenever he anticipated stress.

This is an example of symptoms caused by anxiousness, but not of anxiety disease. With anxiety disease, the symptoms tend to be more severe, are usually intermittent, and often do not show any direct relationship to stress.

Robert was a good example of this. He had episodes of diarrhea, very annoying, unexpected, and at times frightening. On two occasions he was so upset by these symptoms that, unable to reach me immediately, he saw another physician. In both instances he had a full workup, upper and lower gastrointestinal x-rays, gallbladder x-rays, sigmoidoscopy, and stool examination for bacteria and parasites. All tests were negative. These studies had the value of reassuring both of us that there wasn't another problem that had been missed. They had the disadvantage of unnecessary radiation, cost, and of course, inconvenience to Robert. Robert's diarrhea disappeared when his anxiety disease was brought under control with medication.

There is an additional disease process that often seems to be related to anxiety disease called irritable bowel syndrome (IBS). This disease is almost as common as peptic ulcer. It is characterized by periods of intestinal cramps and bowel symptoms, either constipation or diarrhea, or both, alternately. The stools are free of blood, mucus, harmful bacteria, or parasites. X-rays of the bowel are always normal and the bowel lining looks healthy through the sigmoidoscope.

The cause of this troublesome condition is not known, but it seems to occur more often in people who are also suffering from a long-term anxiety disease. Treatment of the irritable bowel syndrome is by dietary precaution and the use of antispasmodic medications, although neither of these is reliably effective. If the person also has an anxiety disease, treatment of that condition helps the IBS as well.

Another annoying symptom, perhaps less common, is gas. Again, this is likely to be unpredictable and is not related to any specific foods. It may be relieved by belching or passing flatus. It is noticed first as a fullness in the abdomen or tightening of the belt. The unpredictability makes this a particularly embarrassing symptom, leading many people to stay home and avoid social situations. While all of the usual remedies for gas may be tried, none is consistently helpful, except for the treatment of the underlying anxiety disease itself.

People who are *anxious* nearly always have eating problems, but these are temporary and disappear after the anxiety has cleared. Whenever I give an after-dinner talk, I am unable to eat. As soon as it's over, I'm very hungry, but, of course, the table has already been cleared. I never seem to have enough foresight to stuff my pockets or hide my plate in the lectern. Or perhaps my foresight has been crowded out by my anxiety.

People with *anxiety disease* usually have persistent eating problems. Some people just can't stop eating—the more anxious they feel, the more they eat. However, most people just can't eat; they have no appetite. While many people do not complain of this symptom, their families report that they "don't eat enough to keep a bird alive." It is not surprising when we consider what is going on in the apparatus with all the gadgets at battle stations ready to deal with the enemy tiger.

The loss of appetite leads to two other very important effects of anxiety disease: weight loss and fatigue. Unexplained weight loss is an alarming finding to a physician and may trigger an extensive, expensive work-up. This may be quite unnecessary. Often the diagnosis of anxiety disease can be made without ruling out all other possible causes. Any testing tends to make anxious people more anxious. They worry about the testing procedure, the outcome, and the possible side effects. Medical studies should always be focused on basic questions, but this rule becomes even more important with anxious patients. It is always worth your while to ask physicians what they are looking for, what the probabilities are of finding something that can be fixed, what happens if the test isn't done, what the side effects and costs are, and whether the test is being done for the physician's legal protection or your own good.

Fatigue that is severe, persistent, and not relieved by a good night's sleep, is perhaps the most pervasive symptom of all in anxiety disease. However, it doesn't have to be present to make the diagnosis of anxiety disease. Some of this fatigue is due to lack of food; the person simply doesn't consume enough calories to have any energy. Some of this fatigue is also due to burning up energy in useless muscle activity like restlessness, pacing, purposeless actions, and increased muscle tension. Sleep difficulties also contribute to making the fatigue a crippling symptom.

We use food in many ways. It has different values and purposes for each of us. It can be a necessity ("you've got to eat to live"), or pure pleasure ("live to eat"), or duty ("eat your vegetables!"), or a cultural or family experience ("like mother used to make"), or a learning experience ("you must at least taste it"), or a punishment ("you bought it, so you eat it"), or a reward ("you may have dessert if you eat everything on your plate"), or even as a tool of seduction (as in the film, *Tom Jones*.) Since food has so many values and meanings to each of us, it is quite understandable that a disorder that affects our eating patterns will have different effects on each of us, and even different effects at different times.

While loss of appetite is the most frequent response to stress, sometimes the opposite symptom occurs. This can be quite bewildering to people. "How can I be gaining weight with everything else that's happening to me?" But often people with anxiety gravitate toward the easier-to-prepare, quicker-to-eat foods such as desserts or candy, which increases the number of calories consumed and therefore increases weight.

People with depression nearly always have eating disorders too, of either too much or too little appetite. Many depressed people use food as a kind of reward. "I think I'll drown my troubles in a Reese's pieces sundae." Since seventy percent of the people with anxiety disease also have depressive symptoms, a disrupted appetite is quite prevalent and unpredictable.

There are two serious eating disorders that should be mentioned—anorexia nervosa and bulimia. Anorexia nervosa is a disease in which a person, usually a young woman, is unable to eat because of a distorted self-image. The victim feels fat in spite of any evidence to the contrary and strives to lose more and more weight. Even the ninety pound thin-as-a-rail person believes herself to be fat, and this delusional fat is totally repugnant to her. It does no good to tell such people or even to prove to them that what they feel is not in agreement with the facts. While this is not an anxiety disease, it provides a good example of what happens in the minds of people with anxiety disease. In other words, proving that there are no snakes in the apartment won't remove the phobic person's horrific fear.

The opposite extreme is bulimia in which a person has an uncontrollable urge to eat, especially sweets. Bulimic people often control their weight by purging themselves after each eating binge.

In *My Name is Carolyn*, a book that describes author Carolyn Miller's personal experience as a bulimic, the opening chapter contains the unforgettably disturbing account of a typical binge. Carolyn, a bright and attractive college student, first sneaks out of her dormitory to avoid being accompanied. She then goes to the drug store and makes a few purchases, but shoplifts a box of laxatives so the clerk won't suspect she has a problem. Next, after gulping an ice cream soda, she buys two bags of chocolate chip cookies. After that she orders a gallon of ice cream with four spoons so that no one will think she intends it all for herself. She hides in an unused basement laboratory, crumbles the cookies onto the ice cream and gobbles it all down. Then she forces herself to vomit.

Both anorexia nervosa and bulimia are accompanied by numerous anxiety symptoms, but they are not forms of anxiety disease, or, as far as anyone knows, caused by anxiety disease. They are usually thought to be caused by deep-seated personality or psychological problems. Both disorders may have extremely serious consequences and sufferers should be urged to have treatment. Surprisingly, just as in anxiety disease, these sufferers do not seek help, perhaps either from a sense of hopelessness or out of shame.

One other symptom associated with the gastrointestinal system is pruritis ani, or rectal itching. This is also likely to be intermittent and can be quite severe. If the itching is not controlled, it leads to scratching, usually furtive but vicious, and can result in deep excoriations or abrasions about the rectum. Occasionally the first symptom of an anxiety disease is the complaint of rectal itching. Also, occasionally I have first noted excoriations on a routine examination and then found out the true cause by asking more questions.

Fortunately, it is usually easy to relieve the symptoms with simple hygiene and the use of over-the-counter cortisone creams. While the symptom is easy to relieve, if the cause is anxiety, it will surely return unless the anxiety disease is brought under control.

Table 4. *Gastrointestinal Symptoms and Some Causes Other than Anxiety*

Symptoms	Other Causes
Dryness of the mouth	Cold medicines, Parkinson's disease, dehydration
Trouble swallowing	Throat infection, muscle weakness, tumor
Heartburn	Spicy foods, hiatal hernia, peptic ulcer, gallbladder disease, food sensitivity
Pain in the pit of the stomach	Peptic ulcer, gallbladder or pancreatic disease
Abdominal cramps	Irritable bowel syndrome, specific food intolerance, infections, food poisoning, worms
Diarrhea	Colitis, infection, worms, overactive thyroid disease
Gas	Irritable bowel syndrome, gallbladder disease, specific food intolerance
Appetite changes	Diabetes, anorexia nervosa, bulimia, any gastrointestinal disease
Rectal itch	Skin allergies, worms

The gastrointestinal symptoms show each of us, even if we didn't know it, our own level of anxiety. While all of these symptoms can be caused by other conditions, the most common cause is anxiety—sometimes anxiousness as a response to stress, and sometimes as a part of an anxiety disease.

As with the skin and respiratory systems, gastrointestinal symptoms can be due to anxiety, anxiety disease, or other causes (see Table 4).

Any of these symptoms—dermatological, respiratory, or gastrointestinal—can happen to any of us when we are anxious. They could also be signs of serious illness, either of anxiety disease or some other disease. Anxiety disease is one of the few ailments that can cause trouble in almost every system of the body, leading to multiple miseries and frequent confusion.

Chapter 7

When the Body Groans

Symptoms of the Musculoskeletal, Cardiovascular, Endocrine, Blood, Urinary, and Reproductive Systems

THE MUSCULOSKELETAL SYSTEM

The musculoskeletal system is the framework of the body and the source of its locomotive apparatus. Without it we would be formless sacks like jellyfish. Ligaments hold our bones, joints, and cartilage together. Tendons attach the muscles, which move the entire body.

While anxiety disease does not have a direct affect on bones, cartilage, joints, or ligaments, its affect on muscles can cause numerous miserable symptoms.

The muscles of the skeletal system have their own specific internal structure, different from the muscles of the stomach, bowel, arteries, or heart. They are operated by the peripheral nervous system, which gives us voluntary control over our muscles. Fortunately, it also contains automatic features. For example, if we wish to wiggle our big toe we can. On the other hand, its usual straightahead neutral position is also the result of muscle action, though it is automatic. We don't have to think about it. The muscles that bend the toe, the flexors, and those that straighten it, the extensors, balance each other automatically, and we don't have to give them a second thought. The muscles in the toes also have a very convenient reflex arrangement, a by-pass to our thought process. If I stub my toe against a hot radiator, the "back off" message goes directly to the muscles. My toe pulls back instantly without my conscious direction.

Muscles make up about forty percent of the body's weight. Each muscle consists of bundles of muscle fibers, each with its own separate nerve. When stimulated by a tiny electrical impulse from the nerve, the fiber contracts. When not stimulated, the fiber returns to its longer resting position.

The muscles are arranged about a fulcrum, or joint. Every joint has two groups of muscles, one going one way, and one the other. To move a bone, one group of muscles contracts and pulls while the other relaxes to allow that movement to take place. Between movements, even at rest, some fibers of each group are contracted, keeping the joint in a steady state.

When we decide to raise a fist to the charging tiger, or better yet, flex our legs and run, we don't have to think about which group does what. We just think "run," and the muscles perform automatically.

The chemicals released when we see or hear the charging tiger or even imagine that we do, cause many body changes, as we have already seen. The purpose of many of these changes is to help the muscles do what they are supposed to do to save us. The heart beats stronger and faster; vessels in the belly constrict to make more blood available for the muscles; digestion stops; breathing quickens to provide us with more oxygen. The elements of the entire musculoskeletal system work in concert, preparing us to fight or run. When we were comfortably stretched out in front of the fire staring at shadows on the cave wall, a few muscle fibers were contracted. With chemical stimulus, such as that from an approaching tiger, our muscles are now activated and ready for action.

But if there is no charging tiger and it was just a nasty figment of our imagination, then all of these muscle fibers have been working in vain, which may have some unhappy results for us. All of this activity, the contraction of these microscopic fibers that make up forty percent of our body, have used an enormous amount of energy, even though we may not have moved at all. This leaves individual muscles exhausted and in a state of severe fatigue.

Severe fatigue after being frightened by a tiger or by the thought of a pouncing tiger seems perfectly reasonable. We know excitement tires us; it's only natural. In anxiety disease, however, the genesis of these reactions may not be so natural or understandable. Often the anxiety feelings surge ahead in the absence of any real or imagined dangers. A person suddenly feels fearful without cause or reason. The body doesn't know better, and responds as though it were in danger or had imagined it: heart and breathing speed up, digestion stops, muscles contract. When the episode subsides, the person is exhausted, and, worst of all, has no explanation—just a feeling of overwhelming fatigue.

When anxiety disease persists, or becomes chronic, the fatigue becomes chronic. The sufferer is exhausted all of the time. This is hard for the sufferer to understand. It is also hard for the family to understand. "How can you be so tired when you didn't do anything? You just think you are tired. You need to get moving and forget about it. No wonder you are tired all the time—you are weak from not moving."

Tiredness, as a medical symptom, can be caused by almost any disease. Usually, with careful history, examination, and testing, the cause can be determined. However, the fatigue of anxiety, or the fatigue of depression, can easily be confused with the symptoms of chronic fatigue syndrome or chronic Epstein-Barr infection. These are terms currently in widespread use describing an ailment characterized by profound and persistent fatigue. There are no conclusive tests to identify this condition, which has been noted most often in young, healthy appearing adults. Since the treatment for it differs from the treatment for anxiety disease, it sometimes requires a prolonged period of close observation to know for sure which is which.

William Roberts made an appointment to see me with only one complaint—severe fatigue. I didn't know him well, having only seen him once or twice in the past. He was in his early sixties and worked in a clerical position with the state government. While he still was able to go to work, he was not functioning well and could barely get his work done properly. He had tried vitamins, Geritol, yeast, and several other remedies suggested by well-meaning family and friends. Nothing worked. He just got more and more tired. My first concern was that he had a malignancy, so I examined him most carefully, asking about additional symptoms. His examination proved normal, as did his blood and urine tests. Since all of this took several weeks, I got to know him better. I realized he was also having many symptoms of anxiety and some depression, although he had not admitted that to himself or to me. At first I thought he was anxious about his health, but soon learned that these symptoms had preceded the fatigue. William didn't think much of my diagnosis of anxiety disease, but was desperate enough to try the medication I prescribed. Over the next few weeks he improved considerably, although I don't believe he ever was convinced of the true nature of his illness.

Within three or four months William was able to discontinue his medication completely. Three years later I saw him again, this time to assist him through the grieving process after the sudden, unexpected death of his wife. They had been walking in a park when she had a fatal heart attack. I was pleasantly surprised that in spite of this stress, his anxiety disease did not recur.

Muscles in a state of useless contraction, the flexors pulling one way and the extensors pulling the other way, can lead to other symptoms as well. When the muscle tension becomes generalized all over the body, the symptoms disperse and the person starts complaining of aching all over. Everything seems to hurt. This is one of the symptoms that bothered Ruth. I had thought that some of her aching was due to early degenerative arthritis, the arthritis of maturity, which is the deterioration of joints that begins to occur in all of us after midlife. As it turned out, much of her muscle discomfort was directly due to the anxiety disease or to the anxiety aggravating her early arthritis. Arthritis is inflammation of the joints. Joints can only move if muscles relax and contract to make this happen. Contracting sore muscles is painful, and moving an inflamed joint is worse. It is easy to see that if the joint is already sore, adding muscle pain to the arthritis pain will exacerbate the problem.

Fibromyositis is another generalized disease of muscle and connective tissue that causes soreness similar to the soreness caused by anxiety disease. Fibromyositis is often chronic, but causes no structural changes as arthritis does. There is a difference, though. Fibromyositis will respond well to aspirin or other anti-inflammatory drugs, but the soreness of anxiety disease won't. However, when the anxiety disease itself is successfully treated, the muscle soreness will disappear.

Sometimes instead of pervading the entire body, muscle symptoms are confined to a single group or region of the body. When this happens the symptoms are likely to be more acute and severe. Headaches serve as a good example. With anxiety disease, some headaches are the result of spasms of the muscles at the back of the neck. These muscles are attached to a sheet of fiber covering the skull that is anchored at the forehead. Tension in these muscles causes pain beginning at the back of the head or at the forehead or both. The muscles sometimes become so tense that they feel hard and sore to the touch. Heat or massage can bring symptomatic relief.

Betty, a woman in her forties, had many problems. She'd had recent surgery for cancer of the uterus; her husband didn't understand her problems or feelings; her daughter's stormy marriage prevented Betty from seeing her only grandchild; she disliked her job as a book-keeper, knew she was making many simple mistakes in entries, and was probably in danger of being fired. Betty also had an inadequately treated anxiety disease that preceded most of these problems. One of her major physical symptoms was severe muscle spasms in her left upper back, neck and shoulder. The muscles were hard to the touch and so tense that there was a visible difference between her two shoulders. This convinced her that she had multiple sclerosis or some other drastic neurological disease. Anti-inflammatory drugs didn't help. Neither did extensive physiotherapy. For two years she experienced some degree of pain and soreness, which at times intensified. Interestingly, her worsen-ing symptoms never had a direct relationship to what was happening in her life. Eventually she accepted the fact that she had an anxiety disease and was able to deal with it with the help of counseling and medication. Although some soreness has still persisted, the flare-ups of severe spasms and pain subsided. Betty had many other symptoms of anxiety, but none so distressing to her as the muscle spasms of her back and shoulder.

One characteristic peculiarity of physical symptoms in anxiety disease is the timing. When we are frightened, we recognize an instan-taneous muscle response: we become startled or jump. The cause–and–effect relationship is obvious. In anxiety disease, it doesn't work that way. The timing of the muscle pain has no apparent correlation to the feelings of anxiety which may come and go. People with anxiety-induced headaches often awake with pain after a sound and restful sleep. Ruth's pain could erupt at any moment or seem incessant; it was unrelated to her anxious feelings. Betty's severe spasms were never related to any events in her life. This irregularity of timing makes it hard for people to recognize that their muscle symptoms are due to anxiety disease.

As in other systems, these muscle symptoms can also result from other disease processes or a combination of anxiety and other diseases (see Table 5).

Table 5. *Muscle Symptoms and Some Causes Other than Anxiety*

Symptoms	Other Causes
Fatigue	Any chronic disease, chronic fatigue syndrome, Epstein-Barr infection, anemia, depression
Generalized aching	Arthritis, fibromyositis, thyroid or parathyroid disease, acute infections
Headaches	Migraine, sinusitis, infections
Regional muscle spasm	Injury or overuse, tendonitis, bursitis

THE CARDIOVASCULAR SYSTEM

The cardiovascular system is the collection of pump and pipes that circulates sustenance throughout the body and hauls off the by-products. Although it sounds like a relatively simple plumbing arrangement, it is not.

This system is controlled by the autonomic nervous system through special nerve fibers that go to each small group of cells. Electrical impulses are carried over this wiring network, but the wires don't actually plug in directly to each component part. Instead, there are special connections, called synapses, that are located between the end of the nerve fiber and its target bit of tissue. A minute gap exists between nerve fiber and cell, and an electrical impulse is carried across this gap by chemicals. These chemicals, formed by special cells in the synapse, are produced in response to the presence of other chemicals, such as adrenalin, circulating in the blood stream. These substances can act to speed up or slow down the electrical charges, producing quick and profound effects on the blood vessels or heart muscle.

The importance of this is that the release of these chemicals is affected by what we see, think, or feel. The same chemicals that prepare our muscles to slay the tiger or run cause the heart to beat stronger and faster.

Over the ages, this design has worked well, but it does have its drawbacks. The heart, in its excited state, may be the source of some worrisome symptoms. In healthy people the heart maintains a fairly steady, even rhythm, varying slightly as we breathe in or breathe out. In most of us there are also occasional missed or extra beats. When stimulated, however, the heart may lose some of its accustomed dependability and have many skipped, extra, or extra vigorous beats. People describe these changes as palpitations.

Ordinarily we don't notice our heart beating. This is amazing since this fist-sized muscle fills and pumps thousands of times each hour and keeps more than six quarts of blood in constant motion. Yet we are blissfully unaware of all of this commotion.

But when there is a sudden change in this activity, we do become aware of it, often in the form of frightening and distressing symptoms. "My heart is going like crazy." "It feels like it's flipping over." "It feels like it's beating on my chest."

Often these symptoms are worse when lying in bed at night, partly because of the physical position of the heart and partly because the distractions of daily living are absent. When I was a new doctor, one of my first home calls was in the middle of the night to see a man who lived in a spooky old farm house in the woods, miles from anywhere. I can remember vividly (probably because of my own anxiety) this man describing his only symptom. "Whenever I sit up, my heart stops." I examined him carefully, but could not find anything abnormal, although he did have a fairly rapid and vigorous heart beat. I gave him a mild sedative and told him to stay in bed until I returned. (I didn't have the courage to have him sit up!)

I realized later that he probably was having palpitations and was suddenly aware of his heartbeat while lying down. When he sat up, he couldn't feel his heart beating against his chest as strongly and thought it had stopped. When I saw him the next day he was up and about. I was greatly relieved; I didn't have to test my theory by getting him up and observing whether or not his heart stopped. He thought I was wonderful—my medicine had cured his heart problem.

Any change in the way our heart beats is a reasonable cause for concern. We know we have only one heart. When there are changes in its rate or rhythm, we are certain that we are in imminent danger. We all know of people who have dropped dead from a heart attack. Naturally we wonder, "Is this how it starts?" "Is this what it feels like?" "Is this happening to me?" "What do I do now?"

A more disturbing symptom is chest pain. Most people know that chest pain is a danger signal and go for help when it happens. Yet in emergency rooms, eighty percent of the people complaining of chest pain do not have heart disease. Even fifty percent of the people in the intensive care unit do not have heart disease. But people with chest pain don't want to hear about percentages and numbers. They are in pain.

"What is happening to me now?" "How can I be reasonable when I'm in pain?" "I need relief, relief from the pain and from the fear that I am about to die of a heart attack."

What is the pain like from a heart attack or heart disease? What other causes are there for chest pain? How can you tell the difference?

The heart is a specialized muscle designed as a pump. The right side collects blood from the circulation and pumps it through the lungs to get oxygen. It then returns to the left side of the heart where it is given a big shove to force it through the rest of the circulation. Since the heart is made of muscle tissue, it needs an ample supply of oxygen, sugar, and other nourishment at all times.

You would think that with thirteen pints of blood flowing through at a rapid rate, without even pausing for a five–minute rest, the heart would soak up everything it needed. This is not the case. The chambers of the heart have a smooth lining, which keeps the blood from sticking and clotting, but does not allow nutrients to soak through. The heart muscle is supplied separately by a group of coronary arteries. A narrowing of these arteries causes the part of the heart muscle that they are supposed to supply, to become ischemic, or lacking in oxygen.

When a muscle does not get enough oxygen it screams for help. If you place a tourniquet around an extremity, it will become very painful within a half hour or so. If you exercise that extremity, as the heart exercises continuously, the pain will occur very quickly.

In coronary artery disease the arteries that deliver oxygen to the heart are partially clogged. If an artery becomes totally blocked, the muscle it is responsible for dies, causing a coronary or heart attack. If this is in a vital area of the heart, or a broad area, the heart can no longer function and the person dies.

When a coronary artery is partly clogged, people are not aware of it unless the heart suddenly needs more blood than can get through the narrowed pipe. When that happens, the body screams in protest causing the pain called angina, or angina pectoris (literally, pain in the chest). Typically, such attacks of pain are brought on by one or more of the three Es: Exertion (climbing stairs), Eating (especially a large or heavy meal), or Emotion (sudden anxiety). The pain disappears quickly when the cause is relieved: the climbing has been stopped, the meal is digested, or the anxious moment has passed. (Or the person can place a nitroglycerin pill under the tongue, which immediately dilates the coronary arteries.) If the cause is not relieved, the affected muscle may die, and a heart attack results.

The pain of angina pectoris usually begins in the left side of the chest. It feels like intense pressure or as if it were being squeezed in a vise. The pain radiates to the left arm and down toward the little finger, or up to the chin. With a heart attack the pain is similar, but persists when the three Es are gone. It is usually accompanied by other symptoms including profuse sweating, nausea, indigestion, shortness of breath, and apprehension. Unfortunately, there are many variations thereof, and at times, for reasons we don't understand, there may be no pain at all. Not having any pain is the worst scenario. When the alarm fails to sound, no precautions are taken.

Anxiety can also cause chest pain. If a person with anxiety disease also has coronary artery disease, the anxiety can cause an attack of angina. This is one of the many reasons why anxiety disease should be treated. Even with a healthy heart, anxiety can cause chest pain, ranging from mild discomfort to severe pain. Along with the pain there may be other symptoms including apprehension, sweating, indigestion, and shortness of breath.

Robert experienced an attack of anxiety that occurred suddenly as a severe pain in his chest with some heartbeat irregularity. Thoroughly frightened, he went to the emergency room, convinced that he was having a heart attack. His heart was fine, but the pain was just as real, just as frightening.

How can you tell the difference between angina pain and anxiety pain? Usually you cannot. When the pain is mild, not directly related to any of the three Es, and you know you are experiencing anxiety, it is probably not angina. Nevertheless, don't bet your life. See your doctor.

Patrick, a man in his thirties, was an only son who had been very close to his father. They shared the same professional office, working together daily. After his father died suddenly of a heart attack at the age of fifty-two, Patrick began having intermittent pains in his left chest. At times it was severe, but never directly related to physical exertion or eating. He had many risk factors for heart disease; he was a heavy smoker, drank alcohol, and was excessively overweight. Yet his basic examination and tests were normal, so I concluded that he was experiencing the heartache of grief.

Still I could not be one hundred percent certain, and could not give the absolute assurance that would have been most comforting given his dangerous lifestyle. As Patrick worked through the grief process, his pain gradually subsided. Now, thirty years later, with no signs of heart disease, and most of the risk factors under control, I can be sure I was right.

The heart is not the only part of the cardiovascular system that reacts to adrenalin. The blood vessels themselves respond by constricting, which causes an immediate rise in blood pressure. Blood pressure is a measure of the blood pressing against the walls of the vessels. If the vessels have narrowed, then the pressure will be higher. This reaction reduces blood loss and guarantees that as long as there is any blood left, the brain and kidneys will get enough to survive. But there is an additional cost. The rise in blood pressure requires the heart to work harder since it is now pumping uphill, trying to force the same amount of blood through smaller tubes.

If anxiety continues, physical changes may occur. Continuous high blood pressure leads to damaged kidneys and arteries in the heart and brain which may lead to a heart attack or stroke. The vessels become damaged by the intense pressure of the blood beating against their walls. Damage to the walls allows deposits of cholesterol to form, building up the plaque and narrowing the vessels even further.

Anxiousness is a sudden, and usually shortlived, feeling. Anxiety disease is a long-term illness, which, if it remains untreated, may affect the body in a long-term way. The chain of symptoms in the cardiovascular system is a vivid example not only of how anxiety disease produces physical symptoms, such as palpitations and chest pain, but how it can lead to physical damage as well. And the damage will lead to more severe symptoms. This is one of the reasons the cause of symptoms may not be either anxiety or heart disease alone but both. It is also one of the reasons for seeking treatment for anxiety disease rather than just putting up with it, or hoping it will go away.

Still many other causes of chest pain exist. After all, many other structures reside in the chest besides the heart and blood vessels, and things can go wrong with any one or combination of them.

Fractured ribs, due to some injury, cause chest pain that is sudden, and grows worse upon taking a deep breath.

When the muscles of the chest wall are strained or injured, pain occurs, but it is usually localized. When you touch the muscles, they feel tender. If you move your arms or twist your body while taking a deep breath, the pain will erupt.

Tietze's syndrome, or costochondritis, also causes chest pain. This condition, of unknown cause, usually occurring in young women, causes pain in the front of the chest and tenderness and swelling of the

Table 6.   *Cardiovascular Symptoms and Some Causes Other than Anxiety*

Symptoms	Other Causes
Palpitations, skipped, extra or irregular beats	Heart disease, excessive use of stimulants (caffeine, tobacco), overactive thyroid
Chest pain	Acute or chronic lung disease, muscle, rib or cartilage disease or injury, esophageal spasm, heart attack, angina

joints between the ribs and the breast bone. Though not a serious problem, it is annoying, but usually subsides by itself after some weeks.

As I mentioned earlier, in the discussion of the gastrointestinal tract, spasm of the lower end of the esophagus can cause pain in the middle of the chest known as heartburn. This has nothing to do with the heart, but can be alarming because of its location. It can be relieved by taking antacids.

Diseases of the lungs can also cause chest pain. These can be sudden, acute problems or more chronic illnesses. Sudden attacks of pain may be caused by blood clots to the lungs or by a sudden collapse of a lung or part of a lung. In either case the person suffers not only pain but severe shortness of breath and severe apprehension. Pain, shortness of breath, and apprehension are also characteristics of anxiety. An examination of the lungs will determine if the person has lung disease. But it does not help us decide whether the person has both lung disease and anxiety, or only one or the other (see Table 6).

THE ENDOCRINE SYSTEM

The endocrine system is a group of small glands located throughout the body that produce hormones, which are secreted directly into the blood stream. It includes the pituitary, islet cells of the pancreas, ovaries, testes, thyroid, parathyroids, and adrenals. The hormones they produce impede, control, or stimulate most other organs of the body.

The pituitary, sometimes called the master gland, is safely nestled in the middle of the head. This location almost guarantees its protection, an indication of how vital it is to our survival. Its hormones are specifically designed to influence other glands. Likewise, it responds to hormones from other glands.

The thyroid gland is located in the front of the neck. Embedded within it are the parathyroid glands, about four, each the size of a grain of rice. The thyroid gland maintains our metabolism and the parathyroids help manage the calcium level. Sometimes the thyroid gland will become overactive, a condition called hyperthyroidism. When this happens the person will experience trembling, nervousness,and palpitations, some of the same symptoms as in anxiety disease. Careful examination will determine the true cause.

Within the pancreas there are groups of cells, known as islet cells, which manufacture and release insulin, essential for our handling of sugar, the basic energy source for all cells.

The sex glands, ovaries in women and testes in men, produce egg cells and sperm. However, they also have an endocrine function, producing hormones to regulate the reproductive activities of the body.

The adrenals are the other principal endocrine glands, and the only ones with a major involvement in anxiety. These are fairly large, as glands go, and can be found sitting on top of each kidney. Each has an outer layer and inner layer of cells, each with a different function. The outer layer produces a group of hormones including cortisone and similar substances that maintain the body's water and mineral balance.

The inner cells produce catecholamines, the most familiar of which is epinephrine or adrenalin. These are the triggers that initiate the chain of symptoms we experience when we become anxious. When the truck came over the hill into our lane, and our eyes were struck with the image, the brain instantly relayed it to the adrenals. We had no time for thinking or analyzing. The reflex poured adrenalin into the circulatory system so we would be ready, at least physically, for whatever happened.

While the function of all of these glands is influenced by the secretions of the pituitary, each gland is also under the direct and immediate control of the autonomic nervous system. Usually there is nothing we can do to increase or decrease their activities. (I said usually, because it is possible through biofeedback to learn to control, or at least influence, some of the activities of the autonomic nervous system.) This inability to control our reactions is important to realize in terms of trying to understand anxiety. We may know that the anxiety we feel is not justified. Your boss is not really going to fire you today; you probably will survive the dentist; and even if you fail your driver's test the world will not end. But knowing all of that doesn't stop the flow of

Table 7. *Endocrine Symptoms and Some Causes Other than Anxiety*

Symptoms	Other Causes
Nervousness, trembling, palpitations	Hyperthyroidism, adrenal tumor, insulinoma

adrenalin or the miserable feelings it causes. We are prepared to attack the boss, flee the dentist, or total the car, whether we intend to do so or not.

These are normal anxieties that are part of life. We all experience them for one reason or another. And we've also learned that a racing heart, flushed face, or the cold sweats will soon disappear and no lasting harm will have been done.

Anxiety disease is different. The symptoms may be the same or much worse. They may disappear quickly or they may persist for long periods of time. Worst of all, they are usually unpredictable. It is one thing to feel anxious when your boss is angry, but a totally different thing to have the same feeling while you are sitting peacefully minding your own business and thinking pure and wonderful thoughts. It is no wonder that people with anxiety disease are often distraught and spend their days looking for answers to unresolvable or nonexistent problems (see Table 7).

THE BLOOD AND LYMPHATIC SYSTEM

The function of the blood and lymphatic system is transportation. The blood carries everything we need to each cell and hauls away the liquid wastes. It also transports special immune cells to attack any hostile invaders. The lymphatic tubes drain away liquid wastes to lymph nodes, which are strategically placed filtering systems designed to destroy any germs. Together this arrangement nourishes us, defends us against injury or disease, and removes waste.

There are no known direct effects of anxiety disease on the blood; however, there could be some indirect effects. Anxiety often causes changes in eating patterns. Sufferers may be unable to eat either because of the physical discomforts of the anxiety or as a result of the shutdown of the digestive system. Others have an insatiable appetite as if they were trying to find solace in food.

In either case, but especially in the former, the changed diet could lead to changes in nutrition and changes in the blood. Anemia, for example, can be caused by a lack of iron or similar nutrients.

While there are no proven ways that anxiety disease affects the lymphatic system, there is evidence that stress can affect it, inhibiting our immune defenses. For example, it has been proven that children from a home in which there is serious marital distress are more likely to get streptococcal throat infections than children in families where there is no major stress.

While a stress response and anxiety symptoms are not the same, there is a possibility that the immune system could also be damaged by sustained anxiety. Family physicians for years have recognized that when mishaps of health occur in a family, one thing seems to lead to another. Many families go through periods when everything goes wrong; one member gets a cold, someone else breaks a bone, someone else gets an ulcer, the kids come down with chicken pox, etc. Everyone feels sorry for them and says it's just bad luck since there is no obvious connection among these misfortunes. But there may be. Anxiety could be one of the connecting links. People who are suffering from anxiety symptoms may be less careful and more preoccupied, which makes them more susceptible to accidents. Also their resistance may be impaired. While this connection is only conjecture now, it is still another argument for why people with anxiety disease should seek help.

THE URINARY SYSTEM

The task of the urinary system is to separate the good stuff from the bad stuff in the blood and get rid of it. The kidneys provide an elaborate filtering system through several miles of very fine tubes. With each heartbeat the arteries pump a large amount of blood through the system. The blood recycles, but the wastewater is collected and stored in the bladder until a convenient and socially acceptable time arrives to eliminate it. The bladder itself is operated by the autonomic nervous system and is not under our control. Fortunately, however, the release valve, or sphincter, and some muscles around the bladder to squeeze it, are under our control.

The urinary bladder reacts to excitement by contracting, causing a sudden urge to urinate. This is a universal experience. Before any public performance there is sure to be a procession of performers going

Table 8. *Urinary Symptoms and Some Causes Other than Anxiety*

ymptoms	Other Causes
requency of urination	Bladder infection, inflammation of the urethra
rgency of urination	Same as above

 and from the rest rooms, reflecting their own personal anxieties at the
oment.

In anxiety disease, symptoms of the urinary tract include a need to
rinate more frequently and more urgently. While inconvenient, these
ymptoms are minor compared with some other more demanding
ymptoms of anxiety. Sometimes, though, they can lead to more serious
roblems.

Edith, the woman who saw more than a dozen physicians, suf-
red unnecessarily because of her urinary symptoms. Because of her
equency and urgency of urination she was treated with an antibiotic
ven though she exhibited no positive evidence of infection. She had a
action to the first antibiotic and was subsequently treated with a
ifferent antibiotic. As a result of these treatments, she developed an
flammation of the colon. While her urinary tract symptoms did
isappear, it was probably not because of the antibiotics. She could have
een spared these additional complications if her underlying anxiety
isease had been recognized and treated successfully (see Table 8).

THE REPRODUCTIVE SYSTEM

The reproductive system functions as a means of procreation and
 a source of great personal pleasure. More than any other system or
ody part, this system involves our deepest feelings, attitudes, and
esires. It affects the feelings, attitudes, and desires of others as well.
his system influences many of our actions, even those so diverse as
electing a mate or buying a car.

Because we are so sensitive to other people's views of our sexuality
nd protective of our own image, we are sensitive to every nuance of
ow our reproductive organs work, or don't work. An occasional
alfunction of the bowels is regarded as a minor annoyance, while a
alfunction of the sexual organs is often perceived as a possible first

sign of decay, the beginning of the end. Because of the sensitivity surrounding this issue, a partner's views or comments may also be grossly misconstrued. Does a bedtime remark, "I have a headache, dear," mean "You are not very appealing to me," or "I'm more interested in someone else," or simply that your partner has a headache. The complicated implications and connotations relating to sex clearly illustrate why sexual functioning may be so easily affected by anxiety.

The organs and areas of the body involved in sexual response are controlled by the autonomic nervous system. Our physical actions, what we do, are part of our voluntary system, but the tissue responses of the lips, nipples, penis, and vagina, are involuntary, and are not under our direct control.

This system would probably work quite reliably, as it does in other animals, if we didn't think about it so much. Along with thinking come anxieties, questions, attitudes, affections—the result of which can make the experience more fulfilling, yet also fragile (see Table 9).

Bert and Polly are a couple in their mid-thirties who have two children. Polly has severe psoriasis for which she has been under constant care but with only partial success. Bert has had a steady job with an accounting firm for more than ten years. Bert and Polly have a good relationship and always had an active sex life. Polly came to see me because she was concerned about why their sexual activity had abruptly ceased, or almost ceased. She was sure that her worsening psoriasis was making her unattractive to Bert.

I asked Bert to come in and he assured me that the problem had nothing to do with his feelings toward Polly but that he neither felt the desire for nor believed that he would be able to have intercourse. He blamed it on his own health problems—intermittent episodes of bron-

Table 9. *Reproductive Symptoms and Some Causes Other than Anxiety*

Symptoms	Causes
Loss of sexual interest	Psychological problems, endocrine disorders
Premature ejaculation	Psychological problems
Impotence	Endocrine disorders, psychological problems, infections in the genitourinary tract
Missed or irregular menstrual periods, excessive menstrual flow, painful menstruation, pain with intercourse	Endocrine disorders

hial asthma, or the drugs he took to control the asthma. Bert had other ymptoms, too, including intermittent abdominal pain, diarrhea, gas, nd depression.

After much more conversation it turned out that Bert was extremely vorried about his job, but had not discussed it with Polly. He had been old by his boss that he would either have to accept a transfer to another ffice out of state, or be fired. His job was apparently highly specialized nd his training was suited for just that specific task. It was the only job e's ever had and he knew that there was no one else locally who would e able to use his skills.

As the story unfolded, I realized that Bert was suffering from all of he symptoms of situational anxiety, technically called adjustment lisorder with anxious mood—an anxiety disease. Adjustment disorder vith anxious mood always has a basis in life experiences, as does osttraumatic stress disorder. The treatment for both of these is counsel-ng or some other form of psychotherapy, with or without help from nedication.

Bert had an anxiety disease because his symptoms interfered with is lifestyle. His is a simple, uncomplicated example.

When he and Polly recognized what was happening to them, they egan planning what to do about his job situation. Once they did so, he anxiety symptoms disappeared.

Both sexual desire and sexual action are powerfully affected by ow we think and how we feel. Anxiety can diminish or eliminate lesire, and it can also interfere with the ability to function sexually. 'hysiological preparation for sex, unlike changes in the other systems, as nothing to do with preparing us for fight or flight.

To the person with anxiety disease, the loss or decrease in sexual lesire is usually not the most prominent symptom. So many other niserable symptoms interfere more directly with daily life that they ccupy the sufferer's full attention.

Loss of sexual desire can be a serious problem for either women or nen, and can be a problem both to the person afflicted and to the artner. In men there may also be additional problems with the ability o have intercourse successfully. This sometimes takes the form of premature ejaculation, where orgasm is reached long before either of the partners wish, resulting in frustration for both.

Jacob and Rose were a couple in their late twenties. I knew Rose well, having delivered her two children, but never got to know Jacob, who rarely accompanied her to the office. About a year after the birth of their second child, Rose made an appointment to talk about a personal problem. With much difficulty she described the sexual problem they were having. Jacob's ejaculation would occur much too soon to provide either of them any pleasure, sometimes even before entry.

Jacob would not discuss the problem with me, except one time briefly by telephone. Rose, however, related a history of many symptoms over a period of several years. These included episodes of smothering sensations, dizzy spells, inability to sleep, tiredness, and worry—worry about everything. From Rose's story, though, I recognized that this was only one symptom of a much larger problem, a long-standing and serious anxiety disorder.

It took Rose almost six more months to convince Jacob that they should get help. They went together to consult a psychiatrist, who used both medication and psychotherapy to control the underlying anxiety disease. After that, their sexual relations improved markedly.

The problem may work in just the opposite way; impotence, or the inability to obtain or maintain a satisfactory erection, may be the cause of stress. This can be frustrating to both partners. The ability to have an erection is not really an ability. It is not under a man's control, as it is dependent on the autonomic rather than the voluntary nervous system. In anxiety disease impotence is likely to be a continuous, rather than an occasional, problem. After a failure at attempted intercourse, the foremost thought in the couple's minds the next time will be the memory of their recent failure. This anxiety frequently assures another failure, generating, in turn, more anxiety.

This vignette—anxiety begets impotence begets anxiety—provides an analogy of what often happens in the progression of an anxiety disease. Anxiety begins, through no one's fault, causing a cluster of symptoms, which the victim does not understand, and which thereby begets more symptoms. If these symptoms are not recognized or understood, they will continue to grow and involve still other systems.

Anxiety disease, I believe, may be one of the major causes for the trouble people have in relating to one another. Herbert, a man in his mid-sixties, was openly gay. He had been in a monogamous relationship for about five years, not quite long enough to precede the AIDS epidemic. He had lost several friends and many acquaintances to the disease. Even though he fully trusted his partner, and in spite of three negative HIV tests, he was increasingly anxious about contracting AIDS. Although he knew his anxiety was out of proportion to any real danger, he could not control it. He recognized that he was becoming increasgly irritated and testy with his friends and business acquaintances. He came to me for help when he realized that he was also destroying his relationship with his lover.

While anxiety symptoms can lead to misunderstandings, it is also true that misunderstandings can lead to anxious feelings. When someone is uncertain about the genesis of the problems, an interpreter may be helpful, be it a family physician, a psychologist, or some other outside caring person, to help sort things out.

Anxiety can also affect the female reproductive system, resulting in missed or irregular menstrual periods, painful menstruation, excessive menstrual bleeding, or pain during intercourse.

There is possibly another intriguing effect of anxiety upon the reproductive system. Couples who desperately want children and are unable to conceive often undergo extensive studies and elaborate procedures to try to overcome their problem. This approach is frequently successful and worth all the effort. Sometimes, though, these efforts fail and the couple decides to adopt a child instead. It has long been observed that, frequently, when this happens, the adoptive mother becomes pregnant. The adopted child seems to prime the pump. This raises the amazing possibility that perhaps the anxiety, in either or both partners, about becoming pregnant might somehow get in the way of the fertilization process. So far this is only speculation, but it is fascinating since we do know how to treat the anxiety component of an infertility problem.

From ghoulies and ghosties and long leggety
beasties, and things that go bump in the
night, good Lord deliver us!

Scottish prayer

Chapter 8

Know Your Own Anxiety
The Six Types of Anxiety Disease

There are six kinds of anxiety disease, each with its own pattern of symptoms and its own natural course if left untreated. In two of these diseases the causes are known; in the others they are not. Sometimes one kind of anxiety disease can lead to another, but often that is not the case. There is no regular expected progression of these diseases like a cold leading to bronchitis, which then leads to pneumonia. Furthermore, some people may have symptoms of more than one anxiety disease at the same time.

All six of these diseases share some similar symptoms, anxiety symptoms, which is the reason they are grouped together and called the anxiety diseases. All of them can last a long time; all of them can make the sufferer miserable; and all of them can be treated with a reasonable expectation of either control or cure.

It is important to make a correct diagnosis among these six devilish flavors, because the treatment of each is quite different. Only a few years ago the diagnosis was not so important. The treatment for all of them was mild sedatives and some kind of talk therapy, or psychotherapy, but all this has changed thanks to new research findings.

Our ability to diagnose these six diseases has also changed thanks to the work of the American Psychiatric Association. They have developed a reference manual called the *Diagnostic and Statistical Manual of Mental Disorders*, that establishes the criteria for diagnosing all kinds of diseases that affect the mind. Since it was first published, the *DSM* has undergone several revisions, the most recent in 1987, and is now referred to as the *DSM-III-R*. These guidelines enable doctors to make clear and distinctive diagnoses so that we can be sure we are talking to each other about the same problems when treating people or when conducting research. Before this, all kinds of terms were used for the same diseases and it was impossible to compare notes and learn from each other.

The manual provides a useful set of standards and guidelines that may be followed strictly in a psychiatric setting. However, the criteria are based on experiences of psychiatrists in their practices, which is quite different from primary care. In primary care, which includes family physicians, general practitioners, and general internists, both medical and osteopathic, we tend to see people at a much earlier stage. Psychiatrists usually see people who have first been treated elsewhere and then referred to them. Most primary care physicians treat patients with anxiety disease or depression themselves, rather than referring them to psychologists or psychiatrists. The recognition and treatment of these illnesses is now a basic component of the training of primary care physicians. For this reason we use the criteria of the *DSM-III-R* as guidelines, but not necessarily as rigid rules.

When there are multiple symptoms and a distinctive disorder cannot be identified, the one causing the most misery is treated first.

The different kinds of anxiety disease are:

1. Adjustment disorder with anxious mood
2. Generalized anxiety disorder
3. Panic disorder
4. Obsessive-compulsive disorder
5. Posttraumatic stress disorder
6. Phobias

ADJUSTMENT DISORDER WITH ANXIOUS MOOD

Mr. T. Bailey Elkins was a grocer in a business established by his father more than two decades before. He made a satisfactory living, but ound it increasingly difficult to compete with the larger supermarkets. He wanted to enlarge his store and make it a kind of supermarket, but as he told me, he didn't have the capital to invest. His father died a few years earlier, leaving him the store and a large tract of farm land near town. Recently a developer from out of town expressed interest in buying the land to build condominiums and a discount shopping mall. Mr. Elkins, after consulting with a local realtor, decided that he would ask $6 million for the property.

Mr. Elkins considered himself to be a very healthy person and had little use for doctors. However, his symptoms brought him to my office visibly shaken. His speech was rapid and unsteady. He had trouble organizing his thoughts and spoke in bursts of words. He told me about the recent events in his life and his concern that the property sale might fall through. A series of physical symptoms plagued him, including diarrhea, sweating spells for no apparent reason, and some dull aching pain across his chest.

Mr. Elkins thought these symptoms were probably due to worry about what might or might not happen with the property sale, but he wanted to be sure. As he said, he didn't want to risk getting sick at a time like this. He also thought there might be something he could do to relieve his symptoms while waiting for a final decision.

After examining him I reassured him that I thought he was right, that his symptoms were due to his anxieties. I encouraged him to talk, and he told me the whole story. It turned out that he had not shared most of the story with his wife. "Why should I worry her or get her hopes up when it might not happen?"

Mr. Elkins had an obvious adjustment disorder with anxious mood. This is one of the two kinds of anxiety disease that is always directly related to something that is happening in life. By definition this group of anxiety symptoms occurs during or soon after some life stress, usually within three months. The symptoms are severe enough to interfere with how a person functions either socially or at work. This diagnostic term is used for problems that last a short time, meaning less than six months. If it lasts longer than that it is placed in the category of generalized anxiety disorder.

The kinds of symptoms a person experiences with adjustment disorder run the whole gamut of anxiety miseries. The most common symptoms are nervousness, a fear that something bad is about to happen, a scared feeling, and constant worrying. The person has trouble thinking straight, finds it hard to remember simple things or to make decisions, even about such trivia as what to wear. The person may have trouble sleeping, especially trouble getting to sleep at night. Often there will be a loss of appetite leading to weight loss. To make matters worse there can be indigestion and diarrhea. Mr. Elkins also had some chest pain, a worrisome symptom and probably the one which prompted him to seek help.

Many kinds of life problems can set off an attack of adjustment disorder. The most likely are those that are very personal in nature such as conflict within a marriage or with one's children, the threat of being fired, or the threat of jail. A major financial loss or the threat of such a loss is often a triggering cause. In Mr. Elkins' case it was a fear of losing the chance for a huge profit. Life-threatening illness, either in yourself or in a loved one, is also a common cause.

It has long been recognized that major life events often have direct effects on people's health. In 1967 a team of psychological researchers developed a list of events that commonly occur in American culture. A group of approximately 400 adults was then asked to rank these according to the severity of impact such an event would be expected to have on them. The result is known as the Holmes and Rahe scale and is pictured in Table 10. Even though some of the statements are obviously dated, and each of us would have our own priorities, it is still useful in identifying the various life stresses that may affect our health. Whether the event is positive or negative in nature isn't important; it nevertheless has an impact.

Not every person experiencing a life crisis will suffer from adjustment disorder with anxious mood. We are all different and how we react to these common stressors depends on many things. One big factor is our own past experience with handling crises. Through experience many people learn coping skills that help them deal with future crises. Others may never have had the need to develop these skills and are more susceptible when stress occurs. Crucial assets for support include people to talk to, professionals to consult, spiritual support, and the assistance of special agencies.

Another significant factor is the suddenness of a crisis. It is easier for a family to deal with the death of a loved one who has been ill than one who dies suddenly. For example, Mr. Elkins had been leading a fairly calm, steady, uninterrupted life before this opportunity abruptly appeared. When it did, he kept it to himself, not sharing fully with his wife or anyone else, until his symptoms got out of hand.

If a person with adjustment disorder with anxious mood does not seek treatment, the symptoms will probably go away once the stressor

Table 10. *Holmes & Rahe Rating Scale*[3]

Relative Rank	Life Event
1	Death of a spouse
2	Divorce
3	Marital separation
4	Jail term
5	Death of close family member
6	Personal injury or illness
7	Marriage
8	Fired at work
9	Marital reconciliation
10	Retirement
11	Change in health of family member
12	Pregnancy
13	Sex difficulties
14	Gain of a new family member
15	Business readjustment
16	Change in financial state
17	Death of a close friend
18	Change to different line of work
19	Change in number of arguments with spouse
20	Mortgage over $10,000
21	Foreclosure of mortgage or loan
22	Change in responsibilities at work
23	Son or daughter leaving home
24	Trouble with in-laws
25	Outstanding personal achievement
26	Wife beginning or stopping work
27	Begin or end school
28	Change in living conditions
29	Revision of personal habits
30	Trouble with boss
31	Change in work hours or conditions
32	Change in residence
33	Change in schools
34	Change in recreation
35	Change in church activities
36	Change in social activities
37	Mortgage or loan less than $10,000
38	Change in sleeping habits
39	Change in number of family get togethers
40	Change in eating habits
41	Vacation
42	Christmas
43	Minor violations of the law

Source: Reprinted with permission from Thomas H. Holmes and Richard H. Rahe, The Social Readjustment Rating Scale. *Journal of Psychosomatic Research*, 11:216(1967). ©1967, Pergamon Press, Inc., New York.

disappears. If the stressor does not go away the symptoms may become chronic. Then, instead of adjustment disorder, the person might develop generalized anxiety disorder.

GENERALIZED ANXIETY DISORDER

Generalized anxiety disorder is a more severe illness than adjustment disorder. Its nature is chronic, and over a period of time more symptoms appear, which change from time to time and system to system. Because of the varied and vague nature of the disease, sufferers are often given pejorative labels like "nervous wreck" or "worry wart" or even worse. Unlike adjustment disorder, it is not likely to clear up by itself.

This disease can begin as an adjustment disorder that is not treated and does not just go away. When this happens, the cause can be traced directly to life stresses, since stress is the precipitating factor for adjustment disorder. However, only half of the people with generalized anxiety disorder have unusual life stresses that can be identified as precipitating causes. For the other half, the cause is simply not known.

Generalized anxiety disorder tends to begin early in life, even as early as the late teens or in a person's twenties or thirties. While the course is long, it is also varied with many ups and downs. Sometimes it seems to go away almost completely, but then returns, often with a new set of symptoms. Looking back, I have at times recognized that a patient responded to treatment for one set of symptoms and did not return until the next set of symptoms appeared. I did not recognize the basic cause, generalized anxiety disorder, until the patient had several such episodes.

There are often complicating factors with generalized anxiety disorder, which make it even harder to recognize. Other physical diseases may be present that produce some of the same symptoms. Alcohol use can complicate the picture since it is effective in relieving anxiety on a short-term basis. However, the anxiety symptoms return quickly, and sometimes are made worse by the use of alcohol. When people feel relief, they are prone to continue using alcohol—easily leading to abuse and perhaps to alcoholism.

Typically people who suffer from generalized anxiety disorder are constantly worried. They are worried out of all proportion to the problems at hand, and have felt this way for a long time—at least six months. They are described as being "hyper" or "keyed up" or nervous and perhaps even irritable. In a couple, there is often a pattern, a kind of worry game. One person worries excessively and the spouse overreacts in reverse, acting totally unworried about anything. This, of course, makes matters worse for the worrier. There are things worth being concerned about in any family, and a true worrier worries about why the unworried spouse no longer worries at all.

Another major characteristic of generalized anxiety disorder is its variety of physical symptoms. These may include the whole array of anxiety symptoms, but the most frequent are headaches with muscle tension, excessive sweating, heat flashes, chest pain, and shortness of breath. They are often accompanied by bladder irritability, and abdominal pain and diarrhea. The person tends to be restless and may tremble. Almost always the sufferer is excessively fatigued.

Concentration is a problem. Sometimes an alert doctor's office staff will recognize people with generalized anxiety disorder before they see the physician. The person may have unusual trouble deciding on an appointment, may change the appointment several times, or forget an appointment entirely. Remembering is a problem and patients frequently call after an appointment to ask questions about the advice given to them earlier the same day.

Most people with generalized anxiety disorder have some symptoms of depression, and at times that may be the most prominent symptom. Since most people with a depressive disease also have anxiety symptoms, it is hard to be sure which came first and which to treat first. Fortunately, both usually respond well to treatment.

The *DSM-III-R* criteria for the official diagnosis of generalized anxiety disorder require that other possible causes of these symptoms be ruled out. Each of the physical symptoms can be caused by a variety of other diseases and some conditions can cause the whole pattern. These include an overactive thyroid gland or the overuse of stimulants, especially caffeine. There are also a number of mental diseases that can cause similar patterns of symptoms, including manic-depressive disorder and schizophrenia. Usually a doctor can identify whether or not any of these or similar conditions are present.

The *DSM-III-R* lists four groups of symptoms characteristic of the underlying anxiety disorder:

1. Excessive worry, beyond what could be considered realistic
2. Muscle tension with such symptoms as trembling, headaches, restlessness, and fatigue

3. Overactivity of the autonomic nervous system, which causes excessive sweating, bladder and bowel symptoms, chest pain, flushes, chills
4. General nervousness, person feels on edge, can't concentrate, impatient, startles easily, has sleep problems

Paul had symptoms in at least three of these four categories. He worried excessively about his impending retirement and eventually became depressed. He had diarrhea, bladder frequency, and abdominal cramps. His major symptom, the one that bothered him most, was severe night sweats. He was obviously irritable, both at home and with me. Muscle tension symptoms, however, did not seem to be part of the pattern for him. He did not have excessive aching, fatigue, or trembling.

Edith, my businesswoman friend from out of town, has generalized anxiety disorder. She is a full-time worrier, while her husband is a great example of the exaggerated "Why worry?" response. Edith confesses that she has felt irritable at times although she has had no sleep problems and no particular difficulty in concentrating or in organizing her thoughts. She has had considerable muscle tension with aching and soreness. She also has had some of the autonomic symptoms, especially bladder irritability, abdominal cramps, occasional diarrhea, and a persistent feeling of dryness of the mouth.

The treatment of this illness is very successful on a long-term basis. However, it is a chronic disease requiring compassion from both family and physician.

PANIC DISORDER

In his book, *The Anxiety Disease*, Dr. David Sheehan relates the story of a woman named Maria:

> Suddenly, unexpectedly, for no immediate apparent reason, her body was overwhelmed by a surge of elemental panic. Everything seemed to race out of control before she could collect her mind to cope with the onslaught. . . .
>
> Her mind was so overcome, she could feel her vision go off. Everything faded out and became detached, and her heart felt like it wanted to jump out of her chest. She felt very dizzy and lightheaded. Her balance got unsteady. Her legs turned to jelly. The fluorescent lights seemed intensely bright and she seemed acutely sensitive to noise. As she felt beads of sweat breaking out on her skin, she noticed she was trembling and having

difficulty controlling the shaking. She was also acutely short of breath and the tightness in her chest worsened the urge to gasp for air. She felt that if she couldn't get out quickly, she would surely suffocate.

. . . The sheer terror and mental panic were beyond anything she could relate to. It was as if something really terrible was about to happen, or that she was dying but wasn't ready . . . She had a strong urge to run, but didn't know where or from what.[4]

People who have had panic attacks describe them as the worst thing that has every happened to them. Even people who have experienced the pain of kidney stones or heart attacks say the feelings of panic are worse. They would do anything to prevent another episode.

The distinguishing feature of panic disorder is the attacks. They are completely unexpected and unprovoked with alarming symptoms. These attacks include both physical symptoms, like sweating, shaking, shortness of breath, racing heart, and mental symptoms like dread and terror.

Ruth described an attack she had in the supermarket. It was so sudden and so frightening that she shoved her cart of groceries to one side and ran out of the store. She thought she was going crazy or had lost her mind.

Robert thought his first attack was a heart attack. With his second attack there was no chest pain, but he was drenched with sweat, short of breath, and feared he was about to die.

Panic disorder is the most frequent of the severe anxiety diseases. According to surveys, three to four percent of Americans either have had panic disorder or will have it during their lifetimes. It happens to both men and women, although it is more common with women. It tends to begin at a young age, usually under forty, and has an up-and-down, come-and-go course. Some people have a few attacks and then never have any more.

While the cause of panic disorder is not known for sure, most researchers believe that one of the major causes is chemical, or metabolic. Like other metabolic diseases such as diabetes, it tends to recur in families. If the cause proves to be chemical, this has implications for treatment and possibilities for prevention.

In panic disorder, attacks vary tremendously from person to person and even from time to time with the same person. Maria had a full-blown attack. Ruth had the same sense of terror, but not all of the physical symptoms, while Robert's symptoms were mostly physical. Recently I received a letter from an acquaintance, Joanne, a professional photographer, that illustrates both the variety of possible symptoms and how they can change.

> Dear Dr. Leaman,
>
> Although I have had panic disorder for a long time, I only recently discovered what it was. I had my first attack twenty years ago when I was twenty-one. I went to my family doctor who told me I was suffering from anxiety and prescribed Librium. I took the medication for about a year, then stopped because it wasn't doing me much good. I was still having the attacks.
>
> My symptoms (dizziness, unsteadiness, skipped heartbeats, shortness of breath, tight chest) recurred off and on over the next seventeen years, although less frequently.
>
> Then I developed new symptoms—numbness and tingling in the hands and feet—which I didn't realize were part of the same disorder. I became worried, especially when the symptoms interfered with my sleep and driving. Sometimes the numbness in my hands would awaken me at night, and sometimes I couldn't feel the brake or gas pedal while I was driving.
>
> I went to an internist who did a complete physical with lab tests. He suspected arthritis, myasthenia gravis or multiple sclerosis, eventually ruling out the first two. He recommended I wear cock-up splints on my arms when I went to bed to alleviate the numbness. The lab tests were inconclusive, so he referred me to a radiologist for x-rays, a neurologist for further testing, and a physical therapist for the splints. I decided against the splints. The x-rays showed nothing abnormal. The neurologist performed another battery of tests. He concluded I had nonspecific idiopathic neuropathy, carpal tunnel syndrome, and cubital tunnel syndrome. He suggested I see a psychiatrist for the neuropathy because he felt it was an emotional problem.
>
> At that point I felt that I'd seen enough doctors and would take care of the emotional problem myself. I didn't want to take the chance of being labeled a hypochondriac or worse.
>
> Finally, a friend prodded me into seeing her family doctor. He asked me a lot of questions about my past medical history and my present symptoms, and did a complete physical. He then told me I had panic disorder, and had had it since I was twenty-one. I was surprised and relieved. At last it all made sense.
>
> Yours truly,
> Joanne

Panic attacks may have all of the acute anxiety symptoms including shortness of breath and sensations of smothering. It may manifest itself as dizziness or faintness or an unsteady feeling, along with trembling, shaking, and sweating. You feel like your heart is racing and you may experience palpitations. Some describe an irregular beating or say that their heart is "flipping over." Often there is a choking sensation or lump in the throat. Sometimes pain erupts in the chest or in the abdomen and nausea or gagging ensue. At times a numbness or tingling sensation is felt on the skin, either all over the body or just in specific parts. Frequently there is sweating, chills, hot flashes, or a mixture of all three. Along with all of this is the fear of going crazy, losing control, or even dying.

Many times, especially early in the disease, episodes or spells occur with just a few of these symptoms. These are called limited symptom attacks. They are focused on one system such as chest pain, palpitations, and shortness of breath. Another attack may feature choking, nausea, gagging, and abdominal pain.

As Joanne found out, episodes like these are often misunderstood and misdiagnosed. This is especially true with the first few attacks. Attacks of nausea and abdominal pain can easily be misdiagnosed as a gastrointestinal virus infection. A doctor may only see in retrospect the pattern of what's happening, that the patient is really having a variety of attacks of the same disease, panic disorder.

To make an official diagnosis of panic disorder, according to the *DSM-III-R* criteria, a person must have at least four anxiety symptoms and have four attacks within a month. However, it certainly is not necessary, or even a good idea, to wait until the disease gets bad enough to have an official label before beginning treatment. This is especially true since the symptoms are so miserable and the treatment so successful.

The course of this illness is extremely variable, in how it starts, how it progresses, and in complications. About half of the people begin with limited symptom attacks, the other half with full panic attacks. In a few the attacks stop and do not return. In others they continue but at infrequent intervals. Generally, without treatment, the disease progresses. The limited symptom attacks become full panic attacks; the attacks come more frequently and are closer together. As this happens people will try more and more to avoid anything or any place that seems to bring on attacks or make them worse.

Panic attacks occur more often in public places like a store, mall, restaurant, crowded streets, or while on public transportation. This makes matters worse. The victim feels that "everyone is watching; no one understands what is happening to me or knows what to do; I really might lose control; there is no place to hide until it passes, if I don't die first."

Early in her illness Ruth had several attacks while eating in restaurants with friends. She soon learned to go out and wait in the car while her friends finished eating. Next, of course, she stopped going out to eat and just stayed home.

Staying home is the next stage, or complication, of panic disorder. Since attacks happen more often in public places and feel much worse, the person learns to venture out less and less. At first the busiest, most public areas, like supermarkets or malls, are avoided, especially at rush hour; then church or synagogue; then restaurants. Eventually, even a visit with friends or a walk around the block may be too frightening. This imprisoning misery is called agoraphobia (literally, fear of the market place).

Agoraphobia is a frequent complication of panic disorder. This was surely what happened to Henrietta who could not force herself to go more than a block from her home. Most of us know people who "just don't go out." Some of them do have other problems or simply choose to stay home, but many such people have agoraphobia.

Agoraphobia is quite different from other phobias in that it probably does not occur except as a complication of panic disorder. The good news is that even at this late stage of the disease, treatment offers real hope. But not everyone who has panic attacks develops agoraphobia. Joanne has not during the twenty years of her illness.

Depression is another frequent complication of panic disorder. Repeated frightening attacks, especially if they seem to be increasing, have a demoralizing effect. This is made worse if family and friends have no understanding of what is happening. The combined effect results in depression, feeling blue, down-and-out, exhausted, tearful, worthless, and unable to enjoy simple pleasures.

Fortunately, when recognized, this depression also responds very well to treatment, sometimes with some of the same medications used to treat the underlying panic disorder.

OBSESSIVE-COMPULSIVE DISORDER

Obsessions are unwanted ideas or impulses that keep popping up over and over again. They may be recognized as foolish or irrational or even disgusting, but the thought or image keeps returning anyway. One patient, a woman with two young children, was very disturbed by the recurring thought that she might injure a family member or herself with a kitchen knife. She wasn't aware of any hostile or suicidal ideas, but this thought kept coming back so vividly that she had to stop cooking, and for a while, could not even allow herself to enter the kitchen.

Compulsions are repetitious activities or rituals that are done repeatedly beyond the point of necessity. I have a little compulsive ritual that I follow whenever I put drops in a patient's eyes. When I pick up the vial of drops I check to make sure it says ophthalmic, then I check it again—and then at least once more, perhaps several times before I put in the drops. It's good to be careful, and this is certainly useful, but checking once or twice should be enough. Nevertheless, I am uncomfortable unless I do it at least three times.

I know a writer who compulsively lays out three pens with three different colored inks and a data pad to the right of her desk—before she can start work on her word processor!

Minor obsessions and compulsions are part of everyday life for most of us. They are not only harmless, but often useful. They help us with careful organization, staying on time, cleanliness, and efficiency. People with well-developed compulsions may make conscientious employees. Certainly I would like both my dentist and my neurosurgeon to be a bit on the compulsive side! But while obsessions and compulsions are a part of life, and well within the bounds of what we consider normal, there is a distinct disease called obsessive-compulsive disorder. A recent survey indicated that one-and-a-half percent of Americans had the symptoms of this disease within the six months prior to the survey and that probably two to three percent will have it sometime during their lifetimes. Often the beginnings of obsessive-compulsive disorder can be traced back to the teen years. It is equally common in women and men.

The most important fact to recognize is that this disease does not necessarily begin with our usual everyday obsessions and compulsions and grow into a disorder. It can occur in anyone. In other words, being a bit obsessive-compulsive does not mean that you are more likely than someone else to develop the disease.

How can you tell if you have "normal" obsessions or compulsions or have a disorder? Ask yourself these three questions:

1. How much time do these ideas and little ceremonies take up each day? If it's more than an hour you might want to seek help.

2. How much does it bother you if you are not able to complete your rituals? Do you get severe symptoms of anxiety, symptoms that interfere with your life or comfort?

3. How much do your obsessions and compulsions interfere with your lifestyle, either at home or at work?

If you answer these questions by acknowledging that these ideas and actions do interfere with life as you want to live it or with your comfort, you quite likely do have an obsessive-compulsive disorder. If so, you might get it under control with professional help.

Various types of obsessions and compulsions are possible, but there are some common themes. Often they focus on aggressive thoughts, sex, religion, or the need for order. This last category may result in the continuous checking, counting, or ordering of things. The fear of contamination with dirt, bodily wastes, or chemicals can lead to repeated cleansing, repeated handwashing, showering and changing of clothes.

Billionaire Howard Hughes, described as an eccentric, was said to have had all the signs and symptoms of this disease. It was reported that he was unable to touch door knobs or shake hands without needing to wash his hands immediately afterward. Partly as a result of this, he almost never left his apartment during the last decade of his life. He was labeled as, and perhaps was, an eccentric but this part of his personality most certainly was a disease, not just a weird quirk. This is one of many examples in which we think of people as strange when they may really be suffering from an anxiety disease. They need our understanding and compassion instead of idle curiosity or derision.

Doubt is another disturbing form this disease can take. Doubts relate to simple tasks such as locking the house, being sure the cigarette is out, windows are closed, stove is turned off, etc. These doubts are natural enough and for most of us are relieved by a simple, single check. But people with obsessive-compulsive disorder may need to check and recheck and recheck.

The course of this illness is long and drawn out with the symptoms getting better and worse from time to time. However, newer forms of treatment have provided great hope for full control.

POSTTRAUMATIC STRESS DISORDER

David grew up as a street kid in Brooklyn. He was big, tough, quick with his hands but, underneath, a very gentle and sensitive person. He was drafted during the Vietnam War at the age of twenty-one. After minimal training he was sent with his infantry outfit to Vietnam.

I met David about two years after he returned and was discharged. He was having terrifying nightmares, and awakened, night after night, screaming. He said little about them, although they apparently were repetitive, almost the same nightmare each time. I assumed they were related to his experience in Vietnam, but he refused to talk about the experience except in the most superficial way, even with family and friends. He worked for a while in a warehouse and tried night school. After about three months he quit both and hitchhiked to New Mexico where he joined a commune he had learned about through a friend. The group was small, and totally withdrawn from the rest of society. They welcomed David warmly—he "felt like family" almost at once. With them he was able to share his experiences and found a caring, supportive reception. Because of that support, David felt he was beginning to recover. He stayed with the group for several years, and then returned to our community. He completed his schooling and is now an instructor at the community college. He says he feels like a whole person and believes he has almost fully recovered. He still has an occasional nightmare, but no longer finds them terrifying and no longer awakens screaming.

David had posttraumatic stress disorder.

This is one of the two anxiety diseases that occur only after some identifiable precipitating cause. (The other is adjustment disorder.) Other anxiety diseases are sometimes precipitated by life stress, but often occur spontaneously without any more stress than usual.

Events that are beyond common human experience are most likely to cause posttraumatic stress disorder. These can be natural catastrophes such as hurricanes, earthquakes, volcanoes, or floods. Or they can be incidents of personal violence like accidents, assaults, rapes, incest, torture, or combat. Sometimes the unexpected loss of personal property in a fire or major theft can be a factor.

The kinds of events and stress that ultimately cause posttraumatic stress disorder depend on the person. In some cases the sufferer may experience the event; in other cases the sufferer may only be a witness to the event. Trauma occurring to other people affects some witnesses profoundly, almost permanently, while others may be deeply moved at the time, but not suffer any long-term disturbed feelings.

This disorder can happen to anyone who has experienced a drastic enough trauma. In general, the very young and very old are the least capable of handling disasters well. People who grow up in a nonsupportive or violent milieu are less resilient than others. Symptoms usually begin within six months of the traumatic event. If the trauma is "man made" rather than a natural catastrophe, bitterness and vindictiveness are more likely to be part of the symptomatology.

To our ancestors an attack by a sabre-toothed tiger might have been part of daily life stress, one they learned to cope with as well as we drive in heavy traffic. For me, the tiger would cause extreme anxiety. But I can imagine my ancestors would be equally traumatized by the sight of a bus or airplane gobbling people by the dozens. The difference is in our experience, our knowledge, and in our specific coping skills.

We all have our own backgrounds with different levels of susceptibility and different areas of vulnerability. We all have our own supports, or lack of supports, our own perceptions, our own past experiences, and our own sensitivities. We all have our own thresholds for coping in the many areas we, as humans, may face. Posttraumatic stress disorder seems to be very much like my personal computer reacting to overload. When I expect too much of my computer, it responds with a maze of jumbled numbers and letters making no sense and continues to do so as long as it remembers the overload. Fortunately, it has a short memory and reverts to normal if I give it a brief rest. With people it is not so easy.

In all of our dealings with people suffering from anxiety diseases, we need to remember that we cannot tell how badly someone else hurts by deciding what they "should" feel or how we think we would feel under similar circumstances. The person with posttraumatic stress disorder needs to know that this is an illness that is not rooted in an inadequate personality, wimpiness, lack of faith, or a defect in character.

The symptoms of this disorder usually begin within six months of the precipitating catastrophe, but may be delayed even longer. Symptoms fall into three major categories and the sufferer ordinarily has multiple symptoms in each of these three areas:

1. The event that precipitated this disorder is relived over and over again. This may happen as nightmares, such as David experienced, or persistent ideas that the person is not able to keep out of mind. This inability to concentrate was the reason David could not continue in night school. Even little events or the wrong words can serve as symbols and trigger off the whole

experience all over again. These recurrent ideas are often much more than simple thoughts. They are experienced almost as real events, even while the person is awake and aware, almost like a trance.

2. A second group of symptoms comes from an effort to avoid the reliving experience. The person makes conscious efforts to avoid thoughts, feelings, or symbols that might trigger these memories. It may even take the form of a partial amnesia for the event. In these efforts the person often seems detached, avoids social contact, and may lose interest in outside activities.

3. Sufferers seem continually on edge. They may be irritable, have temper flare-ups and startle easily. They often experience great difficulty in concentrating and frequently have sleep problems, usually difficulty in getting to sleep.

The symptoms themselves can make treatment difficult. The sufferer may deliberately avoid others, including those who could be most supportive. Often there is a withdrawal from society and from the professional help that is available. Even when they still see friends, friends will find it difficult to be genuinely empathetic to people who won't say what's troubling them.

Sufferers of posttraumatic stress disorder will sometimes recover without professional help, as David did, through time and understanding and caring friends. However, this is a very serious illness and usually requires considerable help, often the services of a psychiatrist. With treatment the disabling effects should cease, but the painful memories never disappear.

PHOBIAS

A phobia is a persistent, excessive, and unreasonable fear. This may be fear of an object, such as an animal; an activity, like fear of flying; or a situation, like being in an elevator. A phobia is not a one-time event, like a first plane ride. It is regular, predictable, and dreaded. It is also excessive. It is reasonable to be afraid of a pit bull terrier, but not a puppy poodle. A phobia is not only unreasonable in the views of others, but the phobic person also knows that the fear is unreasonable. Nevertheless, it is just as real.

Phobias are extremely common, although most people do not seek and do not even need treatment. A recent survey estimated that four percent of men and slightly more than twice that many women have had or will have a significant phobia.

While agoraphobia usually is caused by untreated panic disorder, the whole cause of other phobias is not known. Some may come from a sudden traumatic event, either recent or during childhood. A fear of flying may follow the experience of being in an airplane accident or a near accident. Or it might be traced to an episode with a swing in childhood. More often than not, there is no discoverable explanation.

The difference between a benign fear and a true phobia is whether or not it affects how we live our lives. A phobia interferes with our lives and causes us to avoid situations in which the phobia might occur. There are many gradations of phobias. In some people phobias are simply facets of their personalities. A fear of flying is no problem if you don't need to fly. Fear of heights is probably not a problem in Manhattan, Kansas. The distinction between an innocent or nuisance fear and a phobia that is an anxiety disease is the degree to which it affects us. If the person with a fear of flying wants to become a pilot, or if the native of Manhattan, Kansas wants to move to Manhattan, New York, their phobias will pose serious problems. Decision making will be powerfully affected by their fear. Many people would suffer severe anxiety symptoms just thinking about such a change.

I have a friend who has a phobia of lightning. If we are visiting, and there is a storm, we all simply move down to the cellar where he feels more comfortable. If his job required him to work in a skyscraper office, or if he lived in a high-rise condominium, he would probably be miserable whenever there was a storm, or even after hearing a prediction of a storm.

There are two kinds of phobias, simple phobias and social phobias. Simple phobias are fears of specific situations or objects. For example, claustrophobia is a fear of being in a narrow or enclosed space—an elevator, a telephone booth, or small room with the door closed. Many people can tolerate these situations if the door is open. Claustrophobia can be difficult, even impossible, for people who need to have a nuclear magnetic imaging procedure, for example. This is a medical diagnostic procedure, based on magnetism, that requires a person to spend up to half an hour in a long narrow tube, the magnetic field.

Fear of heights is common, but easily managed by avoiding heights or not looking down. Fear of flying is also very common. Some airlines have developed therapeutic courses for people who want to get over their phobia. Mice, snakes, dogs, or even cats are also the source of phobias for many people. Insects, especially spiders, are another common source, exploited in the movie *Arachnophobia*.

One bothersome and potentially dangerous phobia is the fear of blood or injury. In our offices we usually know who feels frightened or anxious about an injection or withdrawing blood. In such people the physiological reaction is a sudden drop in blood pressure and a slowing of the heart rate, resulting in fainting. This is easily prevented by asking people to lie down during the procedure and for a few minutes afterward. The dangerous part is that some people will avoid medical care because of their extreme fear of any medical or surgical procedure that touches their bodies.

Janice was a patient I saw only once. She was in her mid-forties and consulted me because of some minor injuries suffered in an automobile accident. In the course of examining her I found a significant tumor in her abdomen, probably a uterine fibroid. I wanted to do some additional examinations to be certain, but she could not permit me to do so. I told her that the tumor was probably benign and might regress as she got older, but that I would like to re-examine her periodically. She promised to consider that, but was never able to return to the office. I discussed it with her by telephone and offered to examine her at home, but she could not do that either. Through a mutual friend, I learned that she was never able to see any other physician either. Fortunately, the tumor must have been benign.

A woman named Roberta came to see me for the first time because of a toe fracture suffered in a fall on the stairs. She had spent her childhood in Los Angeles where she had experienced an extremely frightening event with a physician, which she never fully described. Ever since that event Roberta was totally terrified by the thought of any kind of medical examination or treatment. She had successfully avoided physicians for sixteen years with only one exception—a blood test needed for her marriage license. In the course of my examination I discovered that she had an abdominal tumor the size of a small pineapple. She also had uncontrolled diabetes.

We had many long discussions and eventually Roberta allowed me to help her learn to control her diabetes, even though this required periodic blood samples, as infrequently as I could comfortably manage. After nearly a year of discussion, she agreed that she would see a surgeon about removal of the tumor. However, she agreed only after I promised that he would not examine her internally until she was already under anesthesia for the operation. The surgeon agreed, the procedure was carried out, the tumor was benign and Roberta has done quite well since. She still loudly protests each request for a return visit, but is able to do all that is necessary to manage her disease.

Roberta and Janice are both examples of people with blood/injury phobias, where the untreated phobia could lead to disastrous consequences.

Agoraphobia, the fear of being in open or public places, is not a simple phobia, but is considered to be a different illness since it occurs as a complication of panic disorder. A simple phobia is one that is an isolated problem, and not part of another kind of anxiety or of any other disease process.

Social phobias are fears of doing something embarrassing in public. These can include not being able to urinate in a public restroom or not being able to write or eat while being observed. They also include fears of performing in public. This is a fear that you will be unable to perform, or speak, or even answer questions coherently. You are afraid that your voice will show how scared you are, that your knees will buckle, that your hands will shake so badly you won't be able to read your speech, or that you will wet yourself. You fear that what you say will not make sense, will be misconstrued or criticized, or that you won't know what to say next.

As a family physician in solo practice in a small town I had little need to speak in public. However, when I became active in the community, I needed to address small groups and committees. I had severe anxiety about making even simple comments to any committee of more than five people. Gradually, over some years, this became easier for me but the anxiety never disappeared.

When I joined the faculty of a major medical center and became department chair, I needed to speak in larger and larger gatherings, including national meetings. I learned that by writing out every possible thing I might want to say, it was somewhat easier for me, but the anxiety was still there. I remember what a great thrill it was, after I made a speech at a national meeting, to have a woman tell me she envied my ability to speak with such ease. She was amazed to hear how scared I had been, but it may have helped her with her own speaking discomfort. My anxiety had been useful. It improved my performance—I had not gone over the top of the anxiety curve. (See Figure 1 in Chapter 3.)

On one occasion, after years of becoming accustomed to the feelings of anxiety when speaking publicly, I had a kind of anxiety attack in the middle of a major presentation. My knees began to shake, my hands trembled, and I could not think what to say next because I could not focus my eyes on the words in front of me. I tried taking a few deep breaths, but that didn't help. The person next to me handed me a glass of water. That was a welcome offer because my mouth was very dry, but I was afraid to pick it up because my hands were shaking. After a few seconds of pretending to have lost my place, I resumed and got through the rest of my talk, although I may have skipped some sections; I'll never know. Afterward, I apologized to friends for my miserable performance and was surprised to find that they were unaware of my discomfort. They knew I had paused, thought I was merely collecting my thoughts or finding my place, and thought no more about it.

This experience taught me a valuable lesson. The discomfort or nervousness that we are extremely conscious of often is unnoticed by our audiences. When I reviewed what I was saying in that talk, I discovered that I was discussing an issue about which I had very strong feelings, but feelings I had never thoroughly explored or discussed with anyone else. This is very typical of a social phobia. Anxiety symptoms are directly related to the circumstances or particular symbols and cues of the social situation you are in. The social situations are the triggers, not the cause. This is unlike panic attacks, which are usually unpredictable and totally spontaneous.

What happened to me is a good example of an episode of stage fright, one of the most common forms of social phobias. This is also experienced as examination fear or performance anxiety. People with this disorder may find themselves dreading each public appearance more and more. A little anxiousness before a performance or feeling "up" for the big game is probably a good thing—it helps us do our best. Too much anxiety, however, puts us over the normal curve and on the downhill side. Instead of the Great Performance we anticipated, we feel like we have had a Humiliating Defeat. When that happens, whether real or only in our own view, the anxiety before the next event can be paralyzing.

The pattern of symptoms in both simple phobias and social phobias is similar. In both there is anticipatory anxiety, meaning anxious feelings whenever the public stimulus is expected. A person with a social phobia would begin feeling anxious if scheduled to be the next speaker. Similarly in simple phobias, simply walking through a rocky area, if you have a fear of snakes, will trigger the reaction. All of the usual anxiety symptoms, including shortness of breath, chest pain, sweating, nervousness, or apprehension, may occur. The basic difference between these two disorders is the stimulus—an object in simple phobias or a situation in social phobias—and the approach to treatment.

In both of these phobias there is also the possibility of depressive symptoms, particularly if the phobia is interfering with a chosen lifestyle and if the person is making no progress in coping with it. Treatment of phobias is not easy, but can be quite effective.

SUMMARY

There are six distinct types of anxiety disease:

1. Adjustment disorder with anxious mood is always related directly to some life stress, and occurs within three months of the event.
2. Generalized anxiety disorder is a chronic disease characterized by excessive worry and physical anxiety symptoms that last longer than six months.
3. Panic disorder is distinguished by attacks that are completely unexpected and unprovoked and produce alarming symptoms.
4. Obsessive-compulsive disorder is characterized by unwanted ideas, impulses or rituals that consume more than an hour a day and interfere with lifestyle.
5. Posttraumatic stress disorder can occur after some traumatic event that is beyond normal human experience. The sufferer will relive the event over and over, and make conscious efforts to avoid anything that will trigger the memories.
6. Phobias, both simple and social, are persistent, unreasonable and excessive fears about objects, activities, situations, or about doing something embarrassing in public, which are severe enough to interfere with one's chosen lifestyle.

Double, double toil and trouble; fire burn and
cauldron bubble.

Shakespeare

Chapter 9

Double Trouble

Anxiety disease sometimes occurs alone in an otherwise healthy person, who has an uncomplicated life and no health problems. More often, it is part of a larger picture, one of several factors in the problem of living. This is one of the reasons most people with anxiety disease are treated by primary care physicians; they are already being treated for other health problems. Three of these special situations deserve more detailed attention, partly because they happen so often and partly because they add greatly to the miseries and the dangers of anxiety disease.

ANXIETY DISEASE AND ALCOHOL

Alcohol Abuse

The use of alcoholic beverages is an accepted way of life for many of us. It is an accepted and even an expected part of many social events and celebrations. Since the use of alcohol is so prevalent, many people who have anxiety disease are also people who drink.

This presents two potential problems. Some medications used to treat anxiety disorders cannot safely be taken with alcohol. This problem can usually be handled by not taking alcohol and pills at the same time, or by avoiding alcohol while undergoing active drug treatment. The other problem is more subtle. On a short-term basis, alcohol is a very effective drug for anxiety. It is readily available, socially accept-able, cheap (compared with drugs and doctors), and it works quickly. A few quick drinks and the anxious feelings disappear; you are ready for a showdown with the marshall. However, the effect is temporary and may be followed by more anxiety and the need for another dose. Addiction is a real threat, and so is just plain overuse, which can cause physical health damage.

The National Institute of Mental Health survey referred to in Chapter 1 that studied the frequency of various illnesses affecting mental health also showed the scope of alcohol abuse in this country. In the six months before the interviews, one and a half percent of the women in a cross-section of society were alcohol abusers or physically dependent on it—in other words, alcoholic. The figures for men were far more startling—nine percent, almost as high as the figures for anxiety disorder.

When the data were used to project the future, they indicated that four and a half percent of women and twenty-four percent of men would have this problem during their lives. That means that right now, of the one hundred people you know best, more than ten, mostly men, probably have an alcohol problem. During their lifetimes you can expect that thirty of them will develop one.

If you use alcohol at all, how can you tell if you need to be con-cerned about becoming alcohol–dependent or an alcoholic? There is a simple test, widely used and accepted as a sensitive indicator to help answer this question, known as the CAGE questionnaire. It takes less than two minutes to complete. Ask yourself the four questions. Be totally honest in your answers (Table 11).

Table 11. *CAGE Questionnaire for Alcoholism*[5]

1. Have you ever tried to Cut down on your drinking?
2. Are you Annoyed when people ask you about your drinking?
3. Do you ever feel Guilty about your drinking?
4. Do you ever take a morning Eye-opener?

Source: Reprinted with permission from J. A. Ewing, Detecting Alcoholism, The CAGE Questionnaire, *Journal of the American Medical Association*, 252:1905–1907 (1984). ©1984, American Medical Association.

Scoring the test is equally simple. If you said yes to any of these questions, it is interpreted as a suggestion of alcoholism and means that you ought to give the possibility serious consideration. Two or three positive answers means that you may be alcohol dependent. Four yes answers almost certainly means you are alcoholic.

Alcoholism is a disease and can be treated successfully at any stage, although it is less painful in the early stages and the outcome is more certain. The more advanced the progression of the disease is, the harder it is for the person to recognize and admit the problem and finally get help.

Similar Symptoms

Anxiety causes such a plethora and variety of symptoms that it is no wonder people often mistake it for other conditions. One of these is the overuse of alcohol.

When Ruth shoved her cart of groceries aside and bolted from the supermarket, glassy-eyed, trembling, flushed, and confused, was she drunk? An observer might have thought so. When I stopped in the middle of my speech, hands shaking, blushing, sweating, confused, was I intoxicated? Was I having the shakes because I was in sore need of a drink? Someone who did not know me might have thought so. When Howard Hughes refused to leave his quarters for years was he too plastered to venture out? An outsider might have surmised so.

Tremulousness, flushing, rapid heart beat, nausea and vomiting, jumbled words, confused thoughts, and forgetfulness are all symptoms caused by too much alcohol. They are also cardinal symptoms of anxiety, especially the acute anxiety of a panic attack.

Withdrawing from society and showing extreme irritability with family and friends (often especially with family and friends) as David did and Howard Hughes did, can be signs of posttraumatic stress disorder or obsessive-compulsive disorder. But those are signs of alcoholism, too. The recurrent nightmares of posttraumatic stress disorder are terrifying. They can also be confused with the equally terrifying delirium tremens experienced by alcoholics. If a person with these symptoms is seen by a physician during a drinking bout, the diagnosis is clear. Often, however, there is only the history of the symptoms and no elevated blood alcohol.

A misdiagnosis can be very damaging. A patient with anxiety disease who is treated as an alcoholic will become more anxious. A person with alcoholism who is treated with some drugs may become much worse. The combination may cause dizziness, nausea, confusion, loss of coordination, and even loss of consciousness. The person with alcoholism who is unrecognized has no chance at all.

Alcohol as Treatment

Alcohol has long been recognized as a quick and effective drug for acute anxiety symptoms. The gunslinger belts down two or three quick ones before he goes to face the marshall in the white hat who usually declines a drink. (He's just as scared, but not allowed to admit it. Only his doctor knows.) Afterward, the whole town has a few drinks to celebrate—and relieve their anxiety about what would have happened if the good guy had lost.

Recently I had the privilege of introducing a high-ranking health official to a prestigious gathering of physicians. As we sat at the head table we had a lively conversation, but I noted that neither of us ate very much. I was too anxious, and apparently so was he. Shortly before the time arrived for his presentation he excused himself to use the rest room. When he returned a few minutes later, he had a strong odor of whiskey on his breath. His speech was not as crisp and his enunciation was not as perfect as before. I doubt if the audience noticed, but I did. Rather than acknowledging and dealing with his social phobia, he chose to use alcohol to mask the symptoms. It is a choice with inherent risks.

Hilda was a very young, recently naturalized, Scandinavian war bride when I first became her family doctor. Her husband, Max, was a big, overpowering, and sometimes overbearing, man. Together they operated a small but successful diner. Local gossip had it that Max had described himself as a restaurateur and Hilda had expected an elegant establishment. They worked hard, the hours were long, and the tension ran high.

While Hilda and Max seemed to get along, the communication between them was never open or equal. As Hilda matured and became more comfortable in her new society, she wanted the kind of marital equality and true partnership that she saw among their friends. This concept was totally beyond Max's comprehension or, even worse, his concern.

In this setting, and with the additional stress of raising two small boys, Hilda developed a succession of symptoms, only later recognized as anxiety symptoms. First there were sexual difficulties, then general nervousness and headaches, then chest pains and palpitations, and choking sensations.

When I recognized what was happening I tried to help her identify and work through some of her daily problems. I did not see her for several years afterward, except occasionally with the boys for minor acute ailments. Each time she would assure me, in answer to my questions, that things were much better.

One time I thought I smelled alcohol on her breath. I made some excuse to examine her eyes with an ophthalmoscope, which requires close face-to-face contact, and confirmed my suspicions. When I confronted her with it she flatly denied it, although she did admit having one or two drinks at bedtime.

The next time I saw her, nearly a year later, she was complaining of fatigue and pain in the right upper quadrant of her abdomen, which proved to be early cirrhosis of the liver. She insisted that she had been honest with me; she only had one or two drinks at bedtime. What she hadn't said was that those two drinks were six ounce glasses of vodka!

Hilda had an anxiety disease. Her response was to abuse alcohol, which led her to become an alcoholic. Hilda had discovered that some of her anxiety symptoms could be controlled with vodka. No more sleepless nights, unless she had to get up to vomit. No more staying irritated at Max, or being wrapped up in worries. She just floated off. Vodka did not help all of her symptoms, though. Her trembling hands while trying to serve, her flushed face, and her fast heart beat seemed to get even worse.

These symptoms were harder for her because she was afraid to come to me for help. She didn't want me to find out about her comforter—vodka. But I did. After some stormy initial resistance, and with little help from her family, she eventually entered a treatment program. The first three weeks were difficult, but she did make a full recovery. Since then she has remained dry, and attends meetings of Alcoholics Anonymous. The intensive counseling Hilda received as part of the rehabilitation process enabled her to confront Max and insist on continuing counseling for both of them. Together they worked out a much better relationship than they'd ever had before.

Alcohol and Other Drugs in Combination

Alcohol is a drug that reacts with many others. Most people know that they should never take medication and use alcohol at the same time without first checking to see if there is a conflict. This is particularly true of some of the best medications available for anxiety disease and depression.

A physician friend of mine flew from the West Coast to New York City for a speaking engagement. Even though he was traveling first class he knew he would have trouble sleeping on the plane, because he always did. He took a sedative, one often used for sleeping problems in people with anxiety disease. Even though he knew of the possible peculiar side effects that could occur if this drug was used in combination with alcohol, he partook of the free cocktails served in first class. When he arrived in New York he felt fine. Later the same day, however, when he was back in the airport waiting for his flight home, he suddenly realized that he had absolutely no recollection of giving his speech. He had to call a friend and ask if he had heard the presentation! (He had, and it was well received.) That drug in combination with alcohol causes a period of amnesia; he still has no memory of the event.

Anytime you are given a prescription, if you think you might want to use alcohol, check first with your doctor, your pharmacist, or a *Physicians' Desk Reference* (PDR).

And if you are using alcohol to relieve your anxiety symptoms, be honest with yourself and with your doctor. There are better, safer, and more effective methods of treatment.

ANXIETY AND DEPRESSION

At times we all feel depressed—it's part of being human. It is such a common feeling that we have many names for it: low, blue, glum, not worth a damn, like nothing, in a funk, or gloomy. Many people have mood swings. They're up for a time, for a few days or weeks, then down for a while. For some people, these mood swings are only slight variations, and are barely noticeable. For others the swings between up and down are wide and affect the way they live their lives. In women some mood swings are related to the menstrual cycle. In a few people it even seems to have something to do with the phase of the moon. In most, it just is. While there's no entirely rational explanation for feeling down, the feelings are temporary and not too severe. It's just a fact of life.

Depressed feelings can also come from discouraging events.

Olson Crick was a small, sad-looking man in his early sixties. Although he had not been my patient, I had treated his wife a few times.

also knew their eldest son had been killed recently, along with a friend, in a highway accident.

When he came to see me, I immediately offered my condolences. He accepted my words but explained that was not why he had come. He was feeling very depressed, "low," he said. Then he told me that his kidney doctor said he might have to go on dialysis soon. But that wasn't the real problem. He told me that his son had been the driver the night he was killed, and that the friend's parents were suing him. But that wasn't the real problem either. Then he told me that his only daughter had been arrested for shoplifting. But that wasn't the real problem either. (By then I was feeling depressed.) Finally he told me that his wife had caught him at a local motel with his girlfriend and since then he had felt so miserable he needed help.

Olson Crick's problem was feeling depressed, and for abundant reasons. Anyone would feel depressed under similar circumstances. Nevertheless, he did not have the disease of depression.

The disease, depression, is characterized by depressed feelings that are out of proportion to the circumstances. These depressed feelings are accompanied by a group of other physical symptoms. These often include sleeping and eating disturbances, chronic pain syndromes (most often headache, backache, or pelvic pain), thoughts of self-destruction and loss of the ability to enjoy simple pleasures. Olson Crick felt severely depressed, but he had none of the other symptoms.

True, these troubles could have caused an attack of the disease, but for unknown reasons, they did not. Mr. Crick needed help to work through his problems and feelings, but the medications used to treat depression as a disease would not have helped him.

Elsie Entwhistle came to see me. She was usually healthy and sports-minded, a teacher of hygiene and girls' sports at the public high school. As she sat by my desk she kept trying to tell me what was troubling her, but each time she did, she started to cry. I tried to help, thinking someone close to her had died or was about to. I asked about her husband, her baby, her family. Each time she said fine and cried some more. I asked about her students, her job, her friends, and finally she managed a little artificial laugh and said, "Everything's fine. That's the trouble." Everything in her world was fine, but she felt miserable. She could not understand her tears "for no reason." This had been going on for several weeks. She tried to hide it, but "when I smile, I just show my teeth." There were no smiles inside.

Elsie was having her first episode of the disease, depression. It began without warning when her life seemed to be all roses. Since it was her first episode, she did not recognize it. Fortunately, the treatment for this illness is excellent and she responded well.

Depression is a specific disease, different in symptoms, cause, and treatment from "feeling depressed." Depressive disease is common. The 1982 National Institute of Mental Health survey of 10,000 people, randomly selected, showed that in the six months before the interview more than ten percent had experienced some kind of depressive disorder. Depression is twice as common in women as in men. During our lifetimes, about twenty percent of us will experience some form of depression that is severe enough to be classified as a disease by the *DSM-III-R* criteria, rather than just considered to be a passing mood.

Still, anxiety and depression are not particularly reflections of our fast-paced, competitive western life style. In 1986 and 1987, a group of British researchers conducted a study in a remote small village in the country of Lesotho in southern Africa. They used the same kind of questionnaire, and same methods used in this country for the NIMH study, adapted for use in the village. More than three hundred fifty native villagers were interviewed. The surprising result was that generalized anxiety disorder, panic attack, and depression, causing the same symptoms as here, were even more prevalent in the village. Clearly, these diseases are not the price of a modern society.

Anxiety Disease: A Cause of Feeling Depressed

Anxiety disease causes many miseries. The physical symptoms themselves are onerous, and the gnawing uncertainty about which symptoms are due to anxiety and which might be due to heart disease, hidden cancer, or AIDS causes continual apprehension. The feeling of fright about unidentified terrors is exhausting. Suffering through all of these symptoms, while looking healthy, can be a lonely experience. "No one can understand how bad I feel inside when I look so well and the tests are all normal." "I can't go on this way and no one seems to understand why I can't go on this way." "If I were only stronger, or could just pull myself together—if I weren't such a wimp—I must think more positive thoughts. . . ." These and a thousand other thoughts keep running through the minds of people suffering from anxiety disease, which is a frustrating, exhausting, and certainly depressing experience.

Seventy percent of people who have anxiety disease also have symptoms of depression. In some, these symptoms begin to clear as soon as the anxiety disease is treated. Others who are subject to a full-blown clinical depressive disease, possibly precipitated by the anxiety disease, find that the depressive disease also requires separate treatment. These people do not fully recover until both diseases are treated.

In other people, lifting the pall of the anxiety disease seems to uncover an underlying depressive disease. This was the story with Paul. He did not fully recover until both diseases were treated.

Anxiety and depressive disease, although they seem different, have many similarities. Both can be initiated by our reaction to life circumstances, and what's going on around and within us. Both can begin spontaneously in a person otherwise hale, hearty, and happy. Since both also generate much distress in their victims and those around them, it is often impossible, and irrelevant, to sort out which came first, the disease or the troubles.

How Do You Tell Anxiety Disease from Depression?

There are many similar and overlapping symptoms in these two diseases, but no urinalysis or blood test can diagnose either of them. However, there are patterns that make it possible to distinguish between them, or at least to know which disease is predominant. Many doctors use several simple scales, or questionnaires, to help make the correct diagnosis. One of these is called the Raskin-Covi Scales. Each of these two scales asks three questions and for each there are five possible answers. While they are simple to use and score, it is best to do it with someone who knows you, since some of the questions ask about appearance (Table 12).

A score of seven or more on either of the two tests means you probably have a disorder and need help. If both scores are more than seven, then the test with the higher score shows the disorder that is causing you the most trouble.

Another tool is the Hopkins Symptom Checklists. The first part (Table 13) lists nine symptoms of anxiety disease; the second (Table 14) lists symptoms of depression. If more of your symptoms fall in one group than the other, that helps identify which is your major illness.

In both disorders there are sleep and appetite disturbances. Yet the pattern for each disease is different. In anxiety disease people tend to

Table 12. *The Raskin-Covi Scales[6]*

The Covi Anxiety Scale

1 2 3 4 5   *Verbal Report*: Feels nervous, shaky, jittery, jumpy; suddenly scared for no reason; fearful, apprehensive; tense or keyed up; has to avoid certain things, places, activities because of getting frightened; finds it hard to keep mind on task.

1 2 3 4 5   *Behavior*: Appears frightened, shaking, restless, apprehensive, jumpy, jittery.

1 2 3 4 5   *Somatic Symptoms of Anxiety*: Unjustified sweating, trembling; heart pounding or racing; trouble getting breath; hot or cold spells; restless sleep; going unjustifiably more frequently to the bathroom; discomfort at pit of stomach; lump in throat.

The Raskin Depression Scale

1 2 3 4 5   *Verbal Report*: Feels blue; talks of feeling helpless, hopeless, or worthless; complains of loss of interest; may wish to be dead; reports of crying spells.

1 2 3 4 5   *Behavior*: Looks sad; cries easily, speaks in a sad voice; appears slowed down; lacking energy.

1 2 3 4 5   *Secondary Symptoms of Depression*: Insomnia or hypersomnia; gastrointestinal complaints; dry mouth; history of recent suicide attempt; lack of appetite; difficulty in concentrating or remembering.

Key: 1—not at all; 2—somewhat; 3—moderately; 4—considerably; 5—very much
Source: Reprinted with permission from *Clinical Neuropsychopharmacology*, L. Covi, and R. S. Lipman, Primary Depression or Primary Anxiety? A Possible Psychometric Approach to a Diagnostic Dilemma, *Clinical Neuropsychopharmacology*, 7:924–925 (1984).

Table 13. *The Hopkins Symptom Checklist[7]*

HSCL symptoms relatively highest in anxious outpatients

1. Feeling afraid you will faint in public
2. Numbness or tingling in parts of your body
3. Heart pounding or racing
4. Trouble getting your breath
5. Having to avoid certain things, places, or activities because they frighten you
6. Spells of terror or panic
7. Feeling uneasy in crowds, such as while shopping or at movies
8. Hot or cold spells
9. A lump in your throat

Source: Reprinted with permission from R. S. Lipman, Differentiating Anxiety and Depression in Anxiety Disorders: Use of Rating Scales, *Psychopharmacology Bulletin*, 18(4):69–77 (1982).

Table 14. *The Hopkins Symptom Checklist*[7]

HSCL symptoms relatively highest in depressed outpatients

1. Feeling hopeless about the future
2. Feeling all the pleasure and joy have gone out of your life
3. Feeling no interest in things
4. Thoughts of ending your life
5. Not getting any fun out of life
6. Crying easily
7. Sleep that is restless or disturbed
8. Feeling you may never enjoy yourself again
9. Feelings of worthlessness

Source: Reprinted with permission from R. S. Lipman, Differentiating Anxiety and Depression in Anxiety Disorders: Use of Rating Scales, *Psychopharmacology Bulletin*, 18(4):69–77 (1982).

have trouble getting to sleep, or staying asleep. In depression the problem is in awakening very early and not being able to go back to sleep. Some people with depression need more sleep than usual, as if they were trying to escape from the painful existence of consciousness.

Anxious people are often too agitated to eat (me, before a speech), while depressed people lose their enjoyment of pleasures and eat out of necessity. Other depressed people, especially those with weight problems, have an insatiable desire for huge quantities of food. This results in increased weight and adds to the depression.

In both disorders there are problems with thought processes: remembering, organizing thoughts, concentrating, and making decisions. It's as if the multiple symptoms of the disease crowd the consciousness so that it does not work well. Anxious people have flights of thought, jumping from one idea to another, often with rapid speech. In depression thoughts drag, coming so slowly and ponderously that they seem to ooze out.

Although the decision-making process is impaired in both, people with anxiety disease may make quick judgments, or act on impulse, only to change their minds later. Depressed people have difficulty making a decision. It's as if they can see all of the possible bad effects but none of the good. So they avoid making any decision at all.

Survival skills are necessary in our society. Simply driving to the mall requires concentration, judgment, coordination, remembering some basic rules, and decision-making skills. Bigger challenges, like

family relationships, financial management, employment, and community responsibilities, all require a far higher level of these skills. Failure
in any of these areas, including a trip to the mall, can have disastrous
effects on ill people and on their loved ones.

A thoughtless or distracted move in the parking lot can cost a life. A
poor decision about a relationship, overspending, or carelessness on the
job are much more likely to occur when thoughts are muddled by
anxiety. These are the unmeasured, and probably immeasurable, potential ill effects of anxiety disease or of serious depression. This is why
people with these diseases need help so that these risks can be mini-
mized.

In both anxiety and depressive diseases symptoms occur relating
to the chest or abdomen. Again the symptoms can be similar, but the
patterns will be different. In anxiety, symptom onset is sudden and
involves rapid action: quick breathing, racing heart, intestinal cramps,
or diarrhea. In depressive disease chronic pain patterns are frequent.
Most often this includes backache, headache, or pelvic pain. The pain
usually has a slow, vague onset—people often can't remember just
when they were without it. While in anxiety disease there is rapid
breathing or hyperventilation, in depression breathing is usually slow
and punctuated with deep sighs. Since the whole apparatus works
slower, constipation is often a problem.

In both diseases sufferers cry frequently. Crying is a normal and
welcome relief for anyone when there are disappointments, hurt feelings, anger, grief, and frustration. It is said that people who cry readily
don't get ulcers. (An exaggeration no doubt, but it makes the point.) In
anxiety and depression people feel irritable and cry frequently because
of their many and changing symptoms, the frustrations they are experiencing, and simply being misunderstood. Most clinically depressed
people cry "for no reason," often several times a day.

The other major symptom, and the one that usually sends people
to a doctor, is fatigue. People become so tired with both of these
diseases that they cannot function. The fact that they and the people
around them cannot understand why makes the symptoms even worse.
We expect to be exhausted after the exercise of cleaning the house or
mowing the lawn or the tension of a long drive in the fog. To be just that
tired without "justification" is exasperating.

When we are tired we all have our routines and remedies that work
for us: an hour in the recliner, a soak in an herb bath, a good night's
sleep, three extra cups of coffee—for me, five minutes lying on the floor

with my feet on a chair. But with anxiety and depression these do not work. Coffee may make the anxiety worse. Extra sleep may make the depressed person feel more worthless. "I'm just a waste of time."

Even though symptoms in anxiety disease and depression are similar and overlapping, there are also distinct differences. The predominant mood of anxious people is fear: fear of another panic attack, fear of the unknown ("What's really wrong with me?"), and unknown fears or terrors with no basis in reason. Although there are also periods of depression, the overwhelming feelings are fear, worry, anxiety, anger, and tension. For people with depression, the overwhelming feeling is one of sadness. They feel worthless, hopeless, and guilty for feeling the way they do.

At times some anxiety disease sufferers will feel that everything about them is unreal, almost as if they were viewing themselves and their whole world from the outside. This is called depersonalization. It is a devastating feeling and lends credence to the belief, "I really am losing my mind," or "I think I'm dying."

While people with depression usually do not experience depersonalization, they do lose interest in the normal pleasures of life and the ability to enjoy them—humor, beauty, sex, food and drink, even the inner warmth of a hug. Their sense of despair may be so great they wish they had never been born, or that they might not awaken in the morning. Often, they think about harming themselves or committing suicide.

Depression is one of the most miserable diseases from which a person can suffer. It is also extremely dangerous, not only because of the risk of suicide, but also, as in anxiety disease, because of the possible consequences of impaired thinking. The person who would really rather be dead is likely to be a dangerous driver.

The physical symptoms of anxiety tend to be different from those in depression. The most persistent ones for anxiety—palpitations, shortness of breath, sweating, flushing, chills, numbness, trembling, lump in the throat, cramping, indigestion, and diarrhea—are less likely in people with depression. Chronic, recurrent, nagging pains such as dull headaches, pelvic pain, and backache are much more common in depression.

Often people with anxiety disease can trace others in the family who have had some kind of anxiety problem. Depressed people also will often have a family history of depression.

Several features help to distinguish anxiety from depression. People with panic disorder often report that exercise, such as running or tennis, makes them feel worse, and may bring on an attack. There is a sound biochemical basis for this. Depressed people, on the other hand, may feel better for a while after exercise. The problem for them is that they have no interest in doing it.

If you think that you have symptoms of either or both of these diseases, some of these distinguishing features may help you understand what is going on inside you. But there are additional characteristics that others, especially those who know you well, might have observed.

People with anxiety disease are jumpy. They move quickly and startle easily. Restless and impatient, they perch on the edge of chairs because they cannot sit still for long. Their speech is rapid, clipped, and a bit louder than others. Other people are often uneasy in their presence.

Depressed people look dull and have little facial expression or animation. They slump in chairs and move very little. Their speech is slow and soft, as if it's just too much of an effort to talk. "Who would want to listen to me anyway?" Again, other people are affected by their presence, feeling depressed themselves after awhile. As physicians, we often use our own feelings as diagnostic cues while interviewing a patient.

Of course, these characteristics are accentuated here to highlight the differences. People with anxiety disease or depression will actually have some features of both to one degree or another. And for some people, these features are simply part of their normal, healthy personality. We are all different. This is one of the reasons it's important to consult with someone who knows you if you feel you are having problems with anxiety or depression.

Why Differentiate Between Anxiety and Depression?

Not long ago, the treatment for both problems was about the same—psychotherapy, or counseling, plus a mild sedative for anxiety and a mild stimulant for depression.

The treatment now is quite specific. Some medications are excellent for anxiety disease, or even for a particular kind of anxiety disease, but ineffective for depression or for other kinds of anxiety disease. Some drugs have both anxiety-reducing and antidepressant properties. Some are useful for depression, but not anxiety. Choosing the right medication, or combination of medications, has taken on paramount importance.

There is also an array of nondrug treatments to consider, either alone or with medication. Choosing the right one, or combination, requires as accurate a diagnosis as possible.

ANXIETY AND THE HEART

Heart disease and high blood pressure are prominent problems in our society. We all know about them, and how they can cause a heart attack or stroke. There are other kinds of circulatory system problems that are also common, but less notorious, including heart failure, damaged valves, disorders of heart rhythm, or clogged arteries.

Since anxiety disease is also common in our society (an estimated thirteen million of us are affected) there are many people who have both anxiety disease and heart disease, simply by chance. However, the fact is that many more people have symptoms of both than can be accounted for by chance alone. Ample evidence exists showing that these two groups of diseases affect each other profoundly. Nearly everyone who has a heart attack feels anxious, and in some it becomes an anxiety disease. In those who already have an anxiety disease, the added anxiety of a heart attack makes them feel even worse. Many people who have anxiety disease, probably most, have some cardiovascular symptoms as part of their anxiety disease. Indeed, anxiety disease itself may be one of the causes of some cardiovascular disorders.

Why Should This Be?

Although much research has been done, and is still underway, no one knows exactly how the physiological changes of anxiety disease can cause physical damage to the cardiovascular system. It is a hard question to study. Many advances in medical science have been made possible by studying diseased conditions in animals. Since animals don't get the same kind of anxiety diseases we do, this method is somewhat flawed.

Some studies have investigated, nonetheless, what happens in an animal's body when it experiences emotional stress. But stress and anxiety disease are not the same thing. For example, one study used a group of dogs, half with normal coronary arteries and half with partially blocked coronary arteries. Each dog was observed as another dog tried to steal its food. As all the dogs became angry, their blood pressure and pulse rate increased rapidly. In dogs with normal coronary arteries, blood pressure and pulse returned to normal and the heart function, measured by electrocardiography, also returned to normal. In the dogs with partially blocked coronary arteries, the blood pressure and pulse also returned to normal, but the electrocardiogram showed prolonged periods of ischemia, or lack of oxygen to the heart muscle. This is the same finding as in people who have angina. It points to the possibility that, if people react the same way, emotional stress might cause prolonged spasm of the coronary arteries. This could be one way that emotional stress causes damage.

We also know that anxiety, from whatever source, sets loose extra catecholamines. Our brains see or feel danger, instruct the adrenals to squirt more adrenalin and similar chemicals into the system, and the whole anxiety response begins. While this response causes immediate changes we can feel, it may also over time cause physical damage to the heart and arteries. Heart beat and blood pressure rise rapidly and the blood vessels to the central organs constrict. None of this is harmful to a healthy person on a short-term basis. But over a long period of time, forcing blood through narrow pipes at a fast rate puts a severe strain on the pump. The inner linings of the arteries themselves may be damaged, allowing deposits to form and partially clog the arteries. In a person who already has a weakened heart or hardened arteries, the additional damage takes place more quickly.

It has been common knowledge for centuries that there must be some direct connection between stress and heart attacks. People, especially men, have heart attacks while being spectators at sports events. A spouse sometimes collapses with a heart attack at a mate's funeral. The emotional stress of the moment, whether good, in the sense of happy excitement, or bad, in the sense of grief, can have the same dire effects. It can precipitate a heart attack, or the pain of angina. The physical effects of anxiety disease can be the same as those from stress; anxiety in itself is a form of additional stress.

Stress is one of the risk factors for heart disease, along with high cholesterol levels, high blood pressure, cigarette smoking, family history, and diabetes. But what is stress? That depends partly on us, and partly on our circumstances. While I don't mind heavy traffic, our hypothetical cave man might find it as stressful as a tiger on the loose would be to me. Who we are also makes a big difference. Some drivers can calmly wind their way along Washington, D.C.'s Pennsylvania Avenue and enjoy the view; for others it is a miserable melee. Since our backgrounds and personalities are different, our response to stressful situations and our response to anxiety will be different.

A report from the Department of Family Medicine at Tel Aviv University was published in 1976 describing the results of a study designed to find out more about the relationship between anxiety, stressful problems, and heart disease. Ten thousand married men in Israel, ages forty and older, were studied. Each man was interviewed and examined at the beginning of the study and then followed for five years. The purpose was to see how many of them developed angina pectoris, and what risk factors might have contributed either to getting or preventing the disease. All the usual risk factors, including cholesterol level and blood pressure, were recorded. The men also were interviewed carefully about three other areas:

1. The degree of anxiety and anxiety symptoms they typically experienced (not necessarily from anxiety diseases)
2. The kind, number, and severity of life problems or stress they experienced
3. The support they received from a loving wife, or the absence of that support

The results of this amazing study revealed that both anxiety levels and general life problems were major risk factors for angina pectoris. In other words, people who either felt anxious, or had problems in their lives that they considered stressful, were more likely to develop angina than those who did not. It was not necessary to have both anxiety and severe problems; either one increased the rate of angina. In those men who had some heart abnormality before the study, the effects of either of these two factors was far greater.

The most remarkable finding of all, and one never before demonstrated in this way, was how the support of a loving wife clearly affects health. The group of men who enjoyed such loving support had less angina than the group that did not, even if they did have anxiety or severe life problems, or both. This study not only helped confirm what was expected: that anxiety and life stresses contribute to heart disease, but has shown us a method of protection or prevention.

In addition to coronary artery disease, which is the most common form of heart disease, other forms of heart disease, especially heart failure and arrhythmias, are also affected by anxiety. Certainly these diseases enhance anxiety symptoms. The mechanisms that cause this are probably similar to the mechanisms that cause coronary artery disease.

There is another, different and intriguing, form of heart abnormality that seems to be related specifically to panic disorder. It is called mitral valve prolapse.

Elizabeth was a twenty-four-year-old medical technician from Australia, who was in this country to learn about high tech blood analyses. She told me on her first visit, almost before she sat down in the examining room, that she was a runner. She ran during her lunch hour, a minimum of three miles each day.

Elizabeth made the appointment because of pain in her left chest. The pain was never severe, and never radiated into her arm or jaw as in angina. It happened most often while she was running, but sometimes stopped while she continued to run, unlike angina, and sometimes occurred while she was just sitting. She had no other chest symptoms except for occasional palpitations, with a few fast or extra heart beats.

After some more questions I learned that Elizabeth also had many other, seemingly unrelated, symptoms. She had lost her appetite, couldn't sleep well, was worried "about every little thing." She had spells when she suddenly felt scared for no reason and would shake and break out in a cold sweat. She admitted to being very irritable with her colleagues at work. Although this had been going on for some months, she blamed it all on being away from home, until the chest pains started. This frightened her.

When I examined Elizabeth's heart I thought I heard a little clicking sound. The heart usually makes a lub-dub sound with each beat. The sound is made as blood is pushed by the heart, first from the right side (to the lungs), then from the left (through the general circulation). The sounds are caused by the rushing of the blood and movement of the valves.

Elizabeth's heart sound was lub-tic-dub. I suspected she had mitral valve prolapse, and asked her to see a cardiologist in consultation, who confirmed my diagnosis. We agreed that she could safely continue to run, and I started her on treatment for her panic disorder.

The mitral valve is the one between the left upper and lower chambers of the heart. It is about the size of a fifty-cent piece and consists of three small leaflets. These leaflets open when the upper chamber, or atrium, contracts and snap shut when the left ventricle, the main and largest part of the heart, contracts. This allows the blood to be pushed from the left atrium, where it is received from the lungs, into the left ventricle, which has the strength to force it through the rest of the circulation.

In approximately four percent of the population, mostly women, one or more of these leaflets tends to sag, or prolapse. This does not usually interfere with the valve's function, but does make that little tic sound between the lub and dub. Most people with this condition have no symptoms at all and are unaware of it until it is found on a routine examination. Because it can occasionally cause more serious problems, it needs to be investigated further, usually by a safe and simple procedure called echocardiography.

The extraordinary part is that many researchers believe that there is a connection between mitral valve prolapse and panic disorder. Some studies have shown that a greater number of people have both mitral valve prolapse and panic disorder than could be expected by chance. There seems to be no evidence proving that the one condition causes the other. Some scientists have suggested that both conditions are caused by abnormalities of the autonomic nervous system.

The importance of this, if proven true, is that it demonstrates another way in which the cardiovascular system and anxiety are often connected.

There are three possible scenarios for this connection between the cardiovascular system and anxiety:

1. Some people have cardiovascular disease with no anxiety disease. Not everyone who gets heart disease gets an anxiety disorder, or even gets upset about it. Some people, especially if their disease is not sudden or life-threatening, take it in stride and have no particular anxiety about it.

Henry, an active farmer, not quite fifty years old, developed unmistakable signs of serious heart disease. I knew what this would mean to his lifestyle and his livelihood and tried to find some gentle way to tell him. Henry listened impassively and then said "Well Doc, it is what it is. You just have to take it as it comes." And he did, without complaint or fear.

2. Some people have cardiovascular disease and anxiety disease.

One of my early patients was an executive named Elsworth Jones. Elsworth had a large sense of his own importance and the need for immediate treatment whenever he was ill. He had coronary artery disease, complicated by being sedentary and overweight, as well as by his heavy smoking and drinking. He also had anxiety disease and developed a panic state whenever he had cardiac symptoms.

Predictably, he had many crises. Also predictably he had someone call me whenever he had any symptoms. At one point I did a simple analysis of my practice and found that he, alone, represented almost twenty percent of my off-hour, night call, and home call emergencies. This was especially frustrating because he stubbornly refused to accept any preventive measures or any care between attacks. (He said he did not want to run up his bill, but that was only an excuse since he didn't pay his bill anyway.)

When he had an attack, it was impossible to tell how much was due to anxiety and how much was due to the coronary artery disease. Once the symptom spiral started—anxiety causing chest pain causing more anxiety causing more pain, shortness of breath, sweating, palpitations causing more anxiety—it continued until the cycle was broken. But with each episode, he did respond to my medication, or my presence or reassurance. He would soon recover and continue his usual ways. Eventually he died during one of his attacks, after twelve years of these frightening episodes.

That was thirty years ago, but I learned some things from Elsworth. I learned that fear is the major reason for people demanding frequent and special care. If antianxiety drugs had been available then, I believe a combination of them along with cardiac medications would have done wonders for both of us.

Most people with heart disease do have anxiety, fear of heart disease, fear of crippling attacks, and fear of death. This is only natural. In coronary care units one of the routine medications for people admitted with heart disease is an antianxiety drug.

In people who have heart disease and severe anxiety symptoms, treatment of both can control most of the symptoms. Preventing the anxiety symptoms may actually prove life saving since anxiety, through the release of catecholamines, can aggravate the heart disease.

Elizabeth, the runner, had both mitral valve prolapse and panic disorder. She was able to seek the cause of her symptoms, instead of denying them, and ask for help. With her panic disorder under control and her valve disease identified and evaluated, she was able to live with both and even continue to run.

Heart disease and anxiety disease are not incompatible, but it is important to know the extent of the heart disease and any limitations it might impose. Also, it is necessary to control the anxiety disease with treatment. Otherwise Elizabeth could have become another Elsworth Jones.

3. Other individuals have cardiovascular symptoms but no cardiovascular disease. Robert is an example of this. He had pain across the

front of his chest, which he thought was indigestion. When it continued he was certain it was a heart attack and went to the emergency room. The symptoms were real and severe, but the underlying disease was anxiety disease, not heart disease. Nevertheless, Robert was right to seek prompt help.

How could the doctor in the emergency room be so sure that Robert wasn't having a heart attack, and that he was simply having "a stress reaction?" Actually we can never be one hundred percent certain—nothing is absolute when dealing with the human body. There is always the possibility of being wrong. However, we can be sure beyond any reasonable doubt if the history is not typical of heart disease, if the physical examination is normal, if the tests are all negative, and if the patient does have the symptoms and physical findings of an anxiety attack. The biggest and most common difficulty arises when the findings are not clearcut, as when the heart shows a slight irregularity, the electrocardiogram is not perfect, or the blood test results are borderline.

Knowing about these borderline findings, just as knowing that doctors can never be one hundred percent certain, may add to your anxiety. But you need to know the whole truth if you're going to cope with anxiety symptoms. No amount of reassurance will help if you cannot believe it. It is far easier to cope with the anxiety of the known than the doubts and fears of the unknown.

Many of our body's symptoms, and its communication with us, can safely be ignored or at least we can postpone our investigation of them. Some anxiety diseases, like simple phobias or an adjustment disorder, can be safely self-diagnosed. But, not so with affairs of the heart.

When our body tells us, with chest pain, palpitations, or shortness of breath, that something might be wrong with the heart, we must take it seriously. Even if the message is garbled or muttered, even if the pain is not the typical viselike left chest pain radiating to the left little finger, or even if the palpitations come and go, or the shortness of breath is not too severe, we need to listen to our body's communication.

There is an enormous variety of possible heart symptoms. Sometimes the pain feels like heartburn or indigestion. Sometimes it radiates to the head or back or right side. Some people have heart attacks with no pain.

Don't bet your life that your body's message is wrong or that you can correctly explain it. For understanding the truth behind your heart symptoms you need an interpreter.

SUMMARY

Anxiety disease can occur alone, in people who have no othe
illnesses or life problems. More often it happens in combination wit
other circumstances, which is why most people with anxiety diseas
are treated by primary care physicians.

Three circumstances need special attention:

1. Alcoholism and Anxiety Disease. The symptoms of anxiet
disease may be similar to the symptoms of alcoholism. People wit
anxiety symptoms sometimes use alcohol to relieve their symptom
This can lead to abuse of alcohol and does not treat the underlyin
cause—anxiety disease. Alcohol can be dangerous in combination wit
other drugs, including those used to treat anxiety and depressio
Check with your doctor before mixing drugs and alcohol.

2. Anxiety and Depression. Depression is a specific disease, diffe
ent in cause and treatment from "feeling depressed." Depression is
common complication of anxiety disease. There are many overlappin
symptoms, but it is possible to distinguish one from the other. This
important because the treatment for each is different.

3. Anxiety and the Heart. Anxiety disease and heart disease affe
each other profoundly. Studies have shown that stress is a risk factor f
heart disease. Mitral valve prolapse, which often is associated wit
panic disorder, demonstrates one of the ways in which the cardi
vascular system and anxiety are often connected. Anxiety and th
cardiovascular system interact in three possible ways:

- Cardiovascular disease with no anxiety disease
- Cardiovascular disease in combination with anxiety disease
- Cardiovascular symptoms without cardiovascular disease

If you have symptoms suggesting heart disease, have the
checked out. Don't bet your life that you can tell the difference betwee
the symptoms of anxiety and heart disease.

Why is this thus? What is the reason for this thusness?

Charles Ferrer Brown, 1834–1867, *Moses, the Sassy*

Chapter 10

Why Me?

It is not your fault. You can get scurvy or sunburn or scabies if you know how and try hard enough. If you do that on purpose, you have every right to feel guilty while the rest of us point our fingers at you. If you get rabies or syphilis or beriberi or lung cancer, there is a chance you contributed to the disease and could have prevented it. But that is not so with anxiety disease. There are no immunizations, condoms, or special diets to protect you.

You did not try to get anxiety disease in the first place, and couldn't if you tried. You did not fail to take proper precautions; it could happen to any of us. There is no reason to feel guilty about having this disease. But if you still do, even after reading this book, maybe you *should* feel guilty for not accepting your blamelessness.

Nevertheless many people do feel that some way, somehow, they are responsible for having an anxiety disease. There are logical reasons for why they believe this. Many of the feelings, concerns, and attitudes that are so much a part of anxiety disease, are exaggerations of everyday thoughts and feelings.

When we were youngsters we learned to overcome our little fears—of dogs, the dark, the boogie man—through the reassurance of our parents and our own developing courage. As adults, everyday worries (Will I be late? Will the roads be icy? Will I be able to pay the rent? Do I have the gout?) are overcome by finding answers and by putting our concerns in realistic perspectives—by coping. Minor physical symptoms, like headaches, cramps, nervousness, diarrhea, are accepted as part of life and shrugged off.

We learn to handle these minor ills as simple unpleasantnesses. We might even look down on those who can't seem to cope as timid, worrywarts, chronic complainers, or just immature. We certainly do not want to be like them or have other people think of us in the same light.

Anxiety disorders are a giant step beyond these normal worries, but they produce some of the same features in magnified form. A little apprehension about going through a tunnel is not the same problem as having cold sweats, uncontrollable shaking, and chest pain when thinking about the tunnel. The phobia is not just a stage of apprehension. It won't go away by being a bit braver. It is not a personality quirk—it is a disease.

Many of the characteristics of anxiety disease have small parallels in everyday living. We have learned to handle these little things. It is natural to think that an extra effort will be the answer to the big problems of anxiety disease. When it doesn't work it is also natural to think that it is our fault; we need to try harder, and think more positively.

Ernie DeWitt was a respected and much beloved high school coach. He developed a moderately severe generalized anxiety disorder with many physical symptoms. Slowly, very slowly, he came to accept that most of these symptoms were due to anxiety disease. He was even more reluctant to accept the fact that he needed help to control his illness. He could not will it away through strength of character or strength of body. Push-ups didn't work and neither did pep talks.

When Ernie finally admitted that he had a disease, that he was not responsible for getting it, and that he needed help, the results were a wonder to behold. His energy returned, he exuded vitality, and his inner peace was contagious. This acceptance itself was a major part of his therapy. He still needed medication, but his acceptance kept him from struggling with himself over whether or not to take the next dose.

Anxiety disease is not your fault. Accepting this and knowing why it's not your fault is the first step in the direction of healing. It is one of the answers that heal.

HISTORICAL NOTE

Anxiety diseases have probably been around as long as there have been people. In 400 B.C. Hippocrates described a patient with anxiety disease. Demosthenes, the great Greek orator, was said to be subject to stage fright.

Sigmund Freud suffered many anxiety symptoms himself. He thought that anxiety was the response of the ego to a threat. The threat could be entirely imaginary, or subconscious, and the response could be triggered by any remotely related symbol.

As recently as 1969 Dr. Claire Weekes, an Australian psychiatrist, published a book called *Hope and Help for Your Nerves*.[9] She used the term "nervous illness" for anxiety disease, and believed it was caused by sensitization, bewilderment, and fear. She described sensitization as an exaggerated reaction to stress, which was then amplified by bewilderment resulting in fear. Although written before modern understanding of anxiety disorders, many sufferers still find the book's description of symptoms and practical suggestions useful.

The anxiety disorders have been viewed as mysterious afflictions for centuries, inviting many explanations. And while we know more now than ever before, there is still much to learn. But we do know that it is not your fault.

CAUSES OF ANXIETY DISEASE

There are two known causes of anxiety disease: biological and psychosocial. Some anxiety diseases are caused mainly by biological factors, others mostly by psychosocial influences. In most anxiety disorders and in most people both causes are operative. This knowledge has greatly expanded our ability to choose the best remedies, which usually involve a combination of treatments.

BIOLOGICAL CAUSES

The evidence of a biological basis as one of the causes of anxiety disease is overwhelming. It is most obvious when examined through four physical mechanisms: anatomy, neurotransmitters, biochemistry, and genetics.

Anatomy

In 1976 researchers discovered that a specific area of the brain is responsible for many of the manifestations of anxiety. The locus ceruleus is a very small structure at the base of the brain. When this is stimulated electrically, at an extremely low level, it causes a sense of fearlessness or carelessness. A slightly higher stimulation causes distractibility and watchfulness. As the charge is increased this changes gradually to wariness, then alarm, dread, anxiety, fear, panic, and terror. There are no other known areas of the brain which elicit the same response.

Neurotransmitters

Nerve cells are almost connected to other nerve cells. Almost, because the connection, called a synapse, is really a space where the fuzzy end of one nerve cell almost, but not quite, meets the fuzzy end of another. The gap is closed by the chemicals called neurotransmitters, which carry electrical charges.

As we saw earlier, some neurotransmitters are manufactured by special cells at the synapse, and some come from other places in the body such as the adrenals. Others are formed by similar cells in the brain. Of these, about one-third come from the locus ceruleus. The other possible source is some form of medication.

One of the neurotransmitters most significantly involved in anxiety disease is gamma-aminobutyric acid, nicknamed GABA. This neurotransmitter, distributed throughout the nervous system, has a special function. It acts as a brake to slow or block electrical discharges. As in many other bodily functions, muscle action for example, forces exist pushing one way and opposing forces exist pulling the other way. The net result is a system of fine control. One possible explanation for anxiety disease is that the neurotransmitter control system goes out of whack—perhaps there is too much pushing or not enough blocking.

An even more intriguing aspect of synapses is their receptor sites. A receptor site is where the neurotransmitter is received, or docked. Neurotransmitter molecules can't swim around and land on any convenient nerve fiber. Each neurotransmitter has its own specific shape, and can only be received by a site of the same shape.

It may help to think of neurotransmitters as a set of keys. The car key will only start the car; it won't open the front door of your house. Neurotransmitters are the same way. GABA will only fit in a GABA receptor site, and GABA receptors will only accept GABA. There are specific sites in thirty percent of the synapses that accept GABA.

In 1977 two groups of researchers made an amazing discovery that formed the beginning of modern understanding of anxiety disease. They identified receptor sites specifically designed to fit benzodiaze-pines, called BZDs. These are a group of drugs that are effective in the treatment of some forms of anxiety disease. There are BZD receptor sites at synapses throughout the body. Not only that, BZD receptor sites have been found in all animals, all the way down the evolutionary scale to the level of the shark. This seems to indicate that these receptors have survival implications for all of us. After all, we animals tend to shed nonessential attachments, like tusks, talons, and tails.

There is a more important question raised by the discovery of these receptors. It implies that the body naturally makes a neurotransmitter for these receptors, one that we have not yet identified. Certainly it seems unlikely that we would evolve with receptors for a drug like Valium, even before it was invented.

For all the other receptors that have been identified in the nervous system there is a specific chemical that fits; for each lock a key has been found. This time, however, we found the lock, but our locksmith chemists have had to build a key that works—the BZDs.

As Charles Ferrar Brown said, "Why is this thus? What is the reason for this thusness?" It seems obvious that there must be some naturally occurring substance in the body that fits that lock, that acts like a BZD. Perhaps it will prove to be a form of BZD or a similar compound. If so, we would expect it to act like the other BZDs, but even better.

The BZDs have a unique function in the body. They enhance the function of the known neurotransmitter, GABA, and make it more effective, thus possibly eliminating one of the causes of anxiety disease. There are many unanswered questions here. How it works, what it means for treatment, and what other drugs might do the same thing are questions as yet unanswered. These questions and others have stimu-lated an enormous amount of new anxiety research.

Biochemistry

Marlin was a student in the College of Engineering at a university a hundred miles from his home. He was in his junior year and considered a Big Man on Campus—high grade point average, first-string linebacker on the football team, and vice president of his class. His mother, a long-time patient of mine, told me he had been sick for several weeks. She wasn't sure what the trouble was, but said he had gone to the student health service three times and was not getting better. She asked him to come home, and he did, driving himself. He went to our Family Practice Center where he was seen by one of our senior residents.

I learned later that he was having episodes of tachycardia, sudden attacks of very rapid heart action, accompanied by feelings of light-headedness, sweating, and some shortness of breath. The resident arranged a suitable battery of tests. When these were normal, she arranged for a Holter monitor, a device that records a continuous ECG reading for 24 hours. When the results of this were also normal she consulted a cardiologist, who recommended more elaborate procedures. The results of these were also within normal limits.

In the meantime, Marlin felt better and the episodes of tachycardia stopped. Even though no one understood why, he seemed to have recovered and his family urged him to go back to school.

Marlin set off the very next day, by himself, in his own car. When he got about twenty-five miles from home he felt he just could not go on and returned home. He tried again on two successive days with the same results. He then came back to the Family Practice Center and asked to see me. He was comfortable with me. We have known each other all his life. I had delivered him and served as his family doctor. He told me much more than he was willing to confess to the resident. These episodes of tachycardia were always accompanied, sometimes preceded, by an overwhelming sense of fear, with trembling and sweating. He would even have trouble talking. But when he was at home, living with his folks, he felt much better and the attacks stopped.

Marlin, the product of a happy home, the mature, well-adjusted BMOC, the linebacker, and future aeronautical engineer, was having panic attacks. I had known for a long time that anxiety disease can affect anyone, that it does not require a childhood of abuse, a tormented adolescence, or a life of uncontrolled stress. This example, though, made it all the more clear that there is a major biological factor in the cause of panic disorder. Marlin's panic disorder was controlled with medication and simple reassurance.

One of the scientific evidences of this fact is the finding that some chemicals can cause panic attacks, but only in susceptible people. A group of people who had no history or signs of panic disease were given sodium lactate intravenously. Nothing happened. They experienced no unusual symptoms, and felt the same as they did before the injections. But when the same dose of the same drug was given to people who had a history of panic attacks, they had a recurrence. Since the same drug caused different responses, it is obvious that there was something biologically different between the two groups.

It is interesting to note that lactate is one of the byproducts of muscle exertion. This may be why some people get panic attacks during or after strenuous exercise.

Panic attacks can also be induced by several other drugs including high concentrations of carbon dioxide. More research is needed, but it is clear that one of the causes of panic attack is some alteration in the body's chemistry.

Genetics

For more than a hundred years we have known that anxiety disease has a tendency to run in families.

Most studies have reported that between fifteen and eighteen percent of people with anxiety disease will have close relatives who also have anxiety disease. People without anxiety disease will report having only a little over two percent of their close relatives with anxiety disease. When sorted out by kind of anxiety disease, the rate for panic disorder among the people with anxiety disease is twenty-three percent, far higher than for the other disorders.

In spite of strong statistical evidence pointing to a genetic factor, there was still the possibility that anxiety disease could be learned or influenced by family lifestyle or environment. So a study was done in Norway with eighty-five sets of identical and nonidentical twins. The results were that anxiety disease is five times more common in identical than nonidentical twins. As a further bit of evidence, sets of identical twins with anxiety disease who had been separated at an early age were also studied. Again, all had anxiety disease. All of which lends further confirmation to the genetic theory.

All of this information about the anatomy, neurotransmitters, biochemical and genetic factors is essential in helping us understand the causes of these diseases. But it may not mean much to the individual. After all, even if someone in your immediate family has an anxiety disease, it is still most likely that you won't get it.

The main message that should come through concerning these biological factors is that getting an anxiety disease is not your fault. And it also helps to know that there are ways to correct these chemical problems.

At the same time we need to recognize that some of the causes of this disease are psychosocial. The good news here is that many psychosocial causes are even more fixable and have better potential for prevention than the biological causes.

PSYCHOSOCIAL CAUSES

This term describes what goes on inside us and around us. Our psyche is who we are, our conscious and unconscious selves. The social part is our interaction with the environment, what is happening now and what has happened in our lives. The psyche functions on the basis of a complex interaction of inherited traits, what we have learned, our psychological make up, and what is going on around us.

In order to understand the complexities of anxiety disorders, we need to try to understand our psyches and how they interact with the environment and each other.

There are a number of theories to explain how our psyches go awry and we get anxiety disease. Fortunately, each one seems to contribute a bit more to our understanding and enhance the effectiveness of our remedies. There are three principal groups of theories: psychodynamic, learning, and developmental.

Psychodynamic or Psychoanalytic Theory

This theory says that there are unconscious thoughts, ideas, or imaginings that generate symptoms of anxiety. These noxious thoughts may begin in childhood from some trauma either real or imagined, like separation, loss, or abuse. These recurrent ideas, or even suggestions or symbols of these ideas, can set off the anxiety response, eventually leading to anxiety disease.

The implications for treatment are that with the help of a psychotherapist you can gain insight into what has happened to you. You learn to identify the thoughts or objects that trigger anxiety symptoms for you. The expectation is that if you recognize these triggers, they may no longer be perceived subconsciously as a threat and therefore no longer set off the anxiety response.

Learning Theory

There is a group of theories based on the assumption that anxiety is something that is learned, rather than strictly inherited, biological, or the result of unresolved childhood problems.

The theoretical scenario goes something like this: Perhaps we had a bad experience as a child such as being frightened by a little dog and we felt anxiety. We then learned that by avoiding that dog we could avoid that anxiety. But the bad experience may still spread or broaden until we become afraid of all dogs. Then we need to restrict our activities even more to avoid triggering this new anxiety.

The theory further contends that if anxiety is learned, we ought to be able to unlearn it. This means that we should make an effort to learn different, more acceptable and healthier ways of coping with the same bad experiences. We learned in the past that by simply avoiding them, we feel okay, but as the bad stimulus expands, we must avoid more and more things in order to stay comfortable. The avoidance, itself, becomes an obstacle to our way of life. We must learn some way other than avoidance to deal with this stress.

Henrietta was my patient who could not leave her home because of "that moving feeling." I do not know the full facts of the beginning of her tragic story, but, if we apply learning theory, it might have gone something like this:

When her fiance left her waiting at the church, she was not only grief stricken but mortified. Henrietta then stayed with her mother in the physical comforts of their home during a prolonged period of grief. As the grief lessened, she ventured into the community again. But, wherever she went, she felt she was the object of attention, whether real or only in her imagination. She could not tell if others felt sympathy, pity, or derision. Even her well-meaning friends might have made clumsy comments or been misinterpreted.

Henrietta soon began having spells of panic when she was in a group—church, theater, club meetings. These spells of sudden unsteadiness, apprehension, shortness of breath, palpitations, flushing, and sweating, were so severe that she had to leave abruptly. These spells so added to her embarrassment that the thought of the next gathering made her nervous and apprehensive. Soon she began avoiding the larger groups, and so avoided some of the attacks. Then, since she felt better at home, she avoided any groups. For a while this also reduced the attacks. However, since she was no longer seen in public, she became an even greater object of attention anytime she went out. Eventually this became much too painful and she simply stayed home.

Henrietta learned to avoid the situations that caused most of her unbearable panic attacks. The price was high, but the attacks were so fearsome that avoiding them was worth any price. She now had a fully developed case of agoraphobia. Any time she tried to go beyond her self-defined limits, she began to get the intolerable "moving feeling," her first sign of an impending panic attack.

If learning theory is correct, then Henrietta might have recovered, at least to a degree, with a desensitization program. She could have received counseling from a psychologist, who would have accompanied her as she gradually learned to venture farther and farther from home. As she did this it would be expected that she would notice fewer and fewer symptoms. Her body would then learn to respond less violently.

Developmental Theory

Developmental theories point out that children experience a series of common fears such as fear of darkness, storms, boogums, and snorklewackers. These begin around six months of age, increasing until they reach a plateau during childhood and then decrease in adolescence. Among the more prominent of these fears is separation anxiety (the trauma of leaving home and family for the first time) or school phobia (the terror of going to school). The theory is that these fears, if unresolved, may be precursors of panic disorder.

Using the same imaginative method we used for Henrietta, let's suppose that Marlin, the Big Man on Campus, might have been scared to go to school when he was young. Perhaps he had a bad experience as BMIK (Big Man in Kindergarten). Perhaps he was called up front to give a report on "My Trip to the Farm," but wet himself in front of the whole class. Obviously he could never face any of them again. So he stayed home, at first with terrible bellyaches and then just because "I don't feel ke it." Eventually he was eased back into school, but he had discovered omething. If things get really bad, he just wouldn't go to school.

As a college student, Marlin seemed to be doing well scholastically, ocially, and in sports. Something, perhaps only a symbol, triggered the ld reaction. It might have been embarrassment at dropping an easy ass, the thought of failing an easy course in public speaking, or of osing the class election. Whatever the cause, whether symbolic, truly hreatening, or entirely due to incomprehensible internal machinations, he old avoidance mechanism was triggered. He just could not go back o school. The only comfortable place to be was at home.

This is a fantasized example of developmental theory in action. It is lifferent from learning theory where the fears are learned from some xperience or event. In developmental theory, some normal fear that hould have been resolved in the process of growing up still lingers and s potent enough to affect your present life.

Adults who suffer from panic disorder often have a childhood istory of school phobias. It is interesting that one of the principal drugs sed to treat panic disorders is also helpful in treating school phobias. This may, of course, be entirely coincidental, but it also may point to a onnection between the two disorders.

CONCLUSIONS

Most anxiety diseases have both biological and psychosocial auses. Be sure you note that with all of the research, the theories, and liscoveries, *none* of them has resulted in pointing a finger at the patient. n fact, if you still need it, there is overwhelming scientific evidence that hows anxiety disease is not your fault.

Six Anxiety Diseases: The Causes of Each
Adjustment Disorder with Anxious Mood

This disorder is common in both adolescents and adults. It is not predictable; no genetic factors are known. The only factor that may be a predictor is the fact of having had the same condition before.

Adjustment disorder begins only during periods of stress, never on ts own. It becomes a disorder, a form of anxiety disease when the symptoms disrupt your life, sometimes becoming incapacitating. The kinds of stressors that might trigger it vary with each of us, but the most common are deep hurts, uncertainties, and personal conflicts. These include the fear of losing your job or the fear of being found out in some major wrongdoing. Health-related problems are another common cause. These can be concern about cancer, fear of becoming helpless, or of imminent surgery. Even with minor surgery people often fear the worst possible outcomes.

The basic cause of adjustment disorder with anxious mood is psychosocial. It is caused by our reaction to stress. The anxiety response to this stress is, of course, biological.

Generalized Anxiety Disorder

Not much is known about the specific cause of this disease. Because it begins gradually, it is hard to pinpoint exactly how or when it started. In most people it begins in the twenties or thirties, occasionally in the teens.

In about fifty percent of the people with generalized anxiety disorder it is possible to identify some especially stressful events that could have been the catalysts. In the other fifty percent no such factor can be found.

The basic cause of generalized anxiety disorder is most likely biological, with psychosocial factors serving as the precipitant cause.

In some people diagnosed with generalized anxiety disease, their history shows that they had some symptoms of anxiety in brief attacks, much like the limited symptom attacks of panic disorder. This may mean that they were misdiagnosed originally. Or it may mean that panic attacks can lead to generalized anxiety disorder. Or it may mean that both diseases are part of the same process. We simply do not know.

Panic Disorder

Much more is known about the cause of this disease than most of the other anxiety diseases, probably because it is so common and has been studied more thoroughly. It usually begins before age forty, sometimes as early as puberty. Seventy percent of the people with panic attacks are women. Fewer than ten percent are over sixty-five. This may be because attacks dwindle as people age—or people may stop complaining about them.

A definite hereditary pattern has been demonstrated and the specific gene responsible has even been identified. This does not mean that if you have panic disorder you must have a close relative with the disease. Nor does it mean that if you don't have panic disorder, but a lose relative does, that you will probably get it. The odds are still in our favor. Panic disorder appears to be primarily caused by some biological disturbance, but may be influenced by both genetic and psychosocial factors. Ruth's panic disorder seemed to be entirely biological in nature; it came "out of the blue." I never was able to find either genetic or psychosocial factors. If we follow my imaginary scenario, Henrietta's problem was entirely psychosocial. Marlin's panic disorder, following the same process, may have been a complication or consequence of an unresolved school phobia.

Panic disorder is no longer a mysterious ailment of unknown cause. We now know at least three causative factors: biological, psychosocial, and genetic.

Obsessive-Compulsive Disorder

We used to think that this disease was both biological and psychosocial in origin. Recent studies, however, show strong evidence that by far the greatest factor is biological.

Both anxiety and obsessions are a result of the activity of neurotransmitters in the brain. In obsessive-compulsive disorder the principal chemical involved is serotonin, which is different from the chemicals in other anxiety diseases. There is an area in the front part of the brain where serotonin receptors are especially prominent. This is the part of the brain responsible for social consciousness and for being aware of time; of knowing the right thing to do and when to do it. Both of these traits are exaggerated in people with obsessive-compulsive disorder. Conversely, people who have had severe damage to this area tend to become sloppy and socially unconcerned.

There is a new research tool called positron emission tomography or PET scanning. A drug to be studied is made radioactive and then injected into the subject. The PET scan will show pictures of exactly where that chemical is working in people. Scans of people with obsessive-compulsive disorder show greatly increased serotonin activity in that same area in the front of the brain.

Obsessive-compulsive disorder is distinct from the other disorders. It neither begins as another anxiety disease nor does it lead to another.

Posttraumatic Stress Disorder

This disorder is all too common. It is estimated that one percent of us will have it during our lifetimes, and fifteen percent of us will suffer from some of the symptoms.

The initiating cause is some terrifying event, beyond the boundaries of usual human experience. Long-lasting anguish, such as from abuse, incest, combat, or capture, may result in longer-lasting posttraumatic stress disorder than if the cause is an acute trauma.

There are some factors known to make a person more susceptible to this disorder. A traumatic, abusive, chaotic, or nonsupportive childhood is especially damaging. A history of emotional instability or difficulty in coping with normal life stresses may also be a factor. The converse is also true. A stable, loving, supportive family, and developing good coping skills can help protect us. But it seems likely that any of us, regardless of our backgrounds, might be susceptible to this disease in the event of an overwhelming personal catastrophe.

Posttraumatic stress disorder is certainly precipitated by psychosocial factors, but there may be both biological and genetic factors as yet undiscovered.

David, the Vietnam veteran, had a history of adequate coping skills and emotional stability as an adult. This surprised me considering his childhood in Brooklyn. He was the second of seven children. His mother, in her own struggles to survive with a violent and abusive husband, could hardly stand having David at home. His father ignored him. His street fights resulted in visible scars and a police record of multiple offenses. His goal in life as a teenager was to leave home and never return. This was exactly the kind of background that can become a factor in posttraumatic stress disorder.

Having a loving, supportive family cannot provide total insurance against this disease. However, it can provide a sense of value, purpose and meaning, and a refuge of inner peace to which a person can return mentally in moments of extreme despair.

Phobias

Phobias are among the most common anxiety disorders. The simple phobias occur twice as often in women as men, but social phobias are equally divided.

Fears of all sorts are part of childhood, indeed, probably a necessary mechanism for survival. A child may need to have a fear of heights to learn precautions against falling. Most children gradually lose these fears as they reach adolescence.

Phobias are thought to be some form of maladjustment that occurs in the development process. Perhaps there was some especially terrify-

ng event like falling from a great height. Or the child may learn that a
arent shares the same fears.

My friend who goes to the cellar during thunderstorms has no
ecollection of any especially frightening event or of similar fears by
is parents. However, we know that painful memories are often uncon-
ciously squelched. Whatever the exact mechanism, it is thought that
hobias have very deep roots and are the result of some malfunction
f the learning process.

The causes of social phobias are more complex, and certainly less
nderstood than simple phobias. Social phobias involve relationships
ith other people, both those we know and those we don't know, as
ell as our perceptions of self. In simple phobias, the person must deal
ith a specific fear of an object, like snakes, or a situation, like riding
 an elevator. In social phobias, however, the person must deal with
ars arising from both conscious and subconscious attitudes, percep-
ons, and feelings. While social phobias have psychosocial origins,
oth biological and genetic factors are part of the background.

CONCLUSIONS

We now know more about the anxiety disorders than we do about
any other ailments, such as the common cold, addictive disease, or
ven osteoporosis. Knowledge about the cause lets us devise treatments
nat work and helps us find ways to prevent recurrence. It may help us
nderstand something about preventing the disease in the first place.

Only a short time ago, within most of our lifetimes, anxiety
isorders were thought to be merely a state of mind. Not understanding
ne causes can lead to bizarre treatments. In 1891 Dr. Gunn recom-
nended "exercise in the cold, cold showers, plasters on the spine and
stimulating preparation of bitters."

In the eighteenth century many English sailors were afflicted with
curvy because of the lack of vitamin C in their diets—and the fact that
o one had yet discovered vitamin C. A keen observer, however, noted
nat while sailors often got this disease, soldiers never got scurvy. The
nswer was obvious—sailors needed to wear uniforms, too. Unfor-
unately, in spite of the good logic, it didn't work.

"The doctor says I have the gout." That diagnosis makes people
nicker—unless, of course, you are the one who has it. Gout conjures
p images of fat English lords sitting by the fire with a foot propped up,

bandaged to ten times its normal size, smoking a pipe, munching on a leg of mutton, and sipping brandy. According to the *Universal Dictionary of Arts and Sciences*, by E. Chambers, published in London in 1738, gout is caused by "a sedentary life, drinking too freely of tartarous wines; irregular living, excess in venery (sex); and obstructed perspiration and a supression of the natural evacuations." Recommended treatment was ceasing these excesses and taking a variety of herbal concoctions.

We now know that gout is caused by an inborn error of metabolism. The body just doesn't handle the chemical purine very well. As a result, purine may collect around joints, like the big toe, and in the kidneys causing trouble—mostly severe joint pain and kidney stones.

Because we understand the cause, or at least what happens to people with gout, we have a much better idea of how to treat it. We have drugs to help the body get rid of purine. We also can help prevent attacks by avoiding foods that are high in purines, including, as the *Universal Dictionary of Arts and Sciences* recommended, "tartarous wines."

In a general way this is what has happened to the anxiety diseases. There was a tendency among us in the medical profession, who should have known better, to snicker at people who had phobias or were afraid of things that were only imaginary. We weren't always sympathetic with patients who were worried when there was no cause to worry, or who did not have "real" diseases.

Now that we have learned about the causes of these miseries, attitudes have changed and so has treatment. Just as with the gout, some of our earlier forms of treatment look foolish, or at least incomplete. We are now able to control the disease and prevent more attacks. Also as in gout, part of the management is in the use of drugs and part is in learning a new lifestyle or new ways of coping with life's problems.

Isn't it great to be living in the time of BZDs and appropriate psychotherapy, instead of the time of cold showers and plasters on the spine?

SUMMARY

Anxiety disease is not your fault. This is one of the answers that heals.

There are two known causes of anxiety disease: biological and psychosocial.

The evidence for a biological basis for anxiety disease is overwhelming. It includes:

- Anatomy. An area of the brain called the locus ceruleus has been proven to cause an anxiety response when stimulated electrically.
- Neurotransmitters. The body has receptors designed specifically to accept a group of drugs known as benzodiazepines (BZDs).
- Biochemical. In people susceptible to panic disorder, a full-blown panic attack can be induced by chemicals.
- Genetic. Anxiety disease tends to run in families. This does not mean that if a close relative has the disease you will get it too. The odds are still in your favor.

Some causes of anxiety disease are psychosocial. There are three principal theories, including:

- Psychodynamic or psychoanalytic. This theory says that unconscious thoughts, ideas, or imaginings may generate symptoms of anxiety. It implies that if you can gain insight into the causes, the anxiety can be controlled.
- Learning theory. This theory assumes that anxiety is something that is learned and can therefore be unlearned.
- Developmental theory. This theory suggests that something went awry in the childhood development process when children normally move from a time of many fears into a time of decreasing fears, adolescence.

Anxiety disease is caused by a combination of biological and psychosocial factors. The causes of each disease are:

- Adjustment disorder with anxious mood is psychosocial in origin. It begins only during a period of great stress.
- Generalized anxiety disorder is biological in origin with psychosocial factors sometimes serving as the precipitating factor.
- Panic disorder is primarily caused by a biological disturbance, but may be influenced by both genetic and psychosocial factors.
- Obsessive–compulsive disorder is both biological and psychosocial in origin.
- Posttraumatic stress disorder is precipitated by an overwhelming experience.
- Simple phobias, where the fear is focused on a specific object or situation, are thought to be a form of maladjustment that occurs in the developmental process. Social phobias, where the maladjustment is based on relationships and self-image, have psychosocial origins stemming from both biological and genetic factors.

Doctor, doctor, can you tell,
What will make my dolly well?

Anonymous

Chapter 11

What Do I Do Now?

People question their health and well being on an everyday basis: "Is something wrong? Is what I am feeling normal or the start of something bad? Do I have an ordinary headache or a brain tumor? Is my foot numb from keeping my legs crossed too long, or have I had a stroke? Am I having indigestion or a heart attack?"

Usually these questions are only half serious thoughts that flit through our minds. But if the headache and numbness persist, or the chest discomfort is different from what we usually feel, we must decide whether to take action or to ignore it.

When symptoms occur that may be due to anxiety, like fear, nervousness, pain, or physical malfunctions, we also need to make decisions. Robert went immediately to the emergency room when he experienced chest pain. Ruth delayed for a long time because she didn't know how to describe what she felt.

Here are some questions that we can ask ourselves to help make up our minds about the seriousness of our symptoms:

1. Could this be dangerous if not treated? What might happen? (Robert knew that chest pain could mean that he was having a heart attack.)

2. Does it seem to be getting better or worse, more or less often? (Ruth's attacks were getting closer together and more frightening.)
3. Does this seem like anything I've heard about or know about? (Paul had no idea what the profuse night sweats were all about.)
4. How can I get relief? Does this interfere with my life as I want to live it? (Mr. Elkins, the almost millionaire, couldn't stand the suspense.)
5. What does another layperson think?

Any symptoms that you know might be dangerous, like chest pain, bleeding, or a lump, should always be checked. Symptoms that are different from anything you've experienced before, or that seem to be occurring more often, or are getting worse are worth a professional opinion. So are any symptoms that *feel* dangerous—like fear of going crazy or fear of dying. And it's always worth going for help when you need relief or simply can't function, like Mr. Elkins.

It's always a good idea to talk things over with someone else to help you decide if you need professional help. Bartenders and hairdressers are often great consultants, experienced and sympathetic. Even better is someone who knows you well, like a family member or close friend. I have observed that people who live alone seem to come to me with symptoms that other people are able to manage entirely within the family.

The answers to these questions will identify many symptoms that can be disregarded. Even if you don't altogether understand the symptoms, if things are not getting worse, interfering with your life, or suggesting something bad, you probably are safe in ignoring them. Many symptoms do go away. With all of the millions of moving parts, continuous chemical interactions, and constant flow of mental energy, it is amazing that we don't feel more of what's going on inside of our bodies. Many of the sensations we do feel and call symptoms, aren't really signals of something gone wrong. They are only an awareness of our moving parts in action. But when they do become a worry, they need an interpreter—self, friend, or physician. Whenever in doubt, call your family doctor and ask.

An ever-present danger we all face and to which some of us are more susceptible than others is called denial. Denial is the ability to convince ourselves, consciously or otherwise, that nothing is wrong when something really is wrong.

A few years ago a family physician, for whom I have great respect, had a major internal hemorrhage while attending a meeting out of town. He was taken to the hospital where a bleeding peptic ulcer was diagnosed, even though he insisted he'd never had any symptoms of a peptic ulcer. Later, thinking back over the previous months, he did remember some symptoms—intermittent pain relieved by food or antacids (he thought he had eaten too much), even nausea and vomiting (he attributed it to another stomach virus going around). Unfortunately, I was that respected physician. However, I'm pleased to add that I made a full recovery and learned a lot about denial. Denial is a dangerous device. We can counter it by learning to listen to our bodies and by sharing our feelings and symptoms with someone else.

The whole question about when or if to get help for anxiety disease was not as important in the past, because most treatments were less successful. Today, effective help is available, safer, and more dependable. So when in doubt, get help. It's not your fault you feel miserable, so there is no reason for you to put up with it.

Each of the six different anxiety diseases has a different course and different complications. When deciding whether or not to get treatment, it's important to know when to ignore symptoms and put off treatment, or when to get help quickly.

SIX ANXIETY DISEASES: WHEN TO GET HELP

Adjustment Disorder with Anxious Mood

If this disorder begins during a time of great stress and the group of symptoms you get are mainly "nervous," such as trembling, apprehension, sweating, and worry, you probably can make your own diagnosis. But if physical symptoms such as shortness of breath, chest pain, abdominal pain, or diarrhea are present, you will need professional help to be sure of what is going on.

The symptoms of this disorder will usually disappear if the cause or the stressor goes away. If the symptoms are interfering with your lifestyle, you will probably want to get help, especially if the stress is not likely to disappear. If the symptoms last more than a few months, there is a danger that this condition will grow into a generalized anxiety disorder.

Treatment offers prompt help and usually consists of a combination of counseling and short-term medication.

Generalized Anxiety Disorder

This disorder, although easily suspected, is never easy to diagnose.

Most people with generalized anxiety disorder have episodes of physical symptoms, often in different systems—cardiovascular, pulmonary, gastrointestinal, and genitourinary. Each episode may appear to be due to causes other than anxiety. Often, by the time the usual battery of tests is completed, the symptoms subside. The correct diagnosis is often suspected only after several months of observation. Because of this pattern, many people have trouble believing that their symptoms are due to an anxiety disease. Paul would have found it easier to believe he had tuberculosis or cancer or even a touch of leprosy.

For this disease you will certainly want treatment and the sooner, the better. With effective treatment, people are often pleasantly surprised to find that many of the physical symptoms they have learned to accept begin to subside—headache, nervousness, recurring diarrhea, abdominal cramps, palpitations, and chest pains.

Without treatment, the disease tends to go on and on, and eventual complications become inevitable. One of the most regrettable is iatrogenic—ill effects from tests or procedures done to determine a physical cause, or from medications or surgery, which try to provide relief from recurrent symptoms.

The other major complication is depression, which occurs in more than seventy percent of people with untreated, or inadequately treated, generalized anxiety disorder.

Usually treatment is quite effective, but requires counseling and long-term use of medications, sometimes for several years.

Panic Disorder

If you recognize the little spells you are having as limited symptom attacks, you might guess you have panic disorder. These little spells would include a few anxiety symptoms that come on for no apparent reason and last only five to ten minutes. I have never known anyone, however, who was able to make this self-diagnosis at such an early stage.

True panic attacks should be easy to recognize. The difficulty is that the attacks are so frightening that a diagnosis of some more mortal condition is more believable than an anxiety disease.

Without treatment this disease sometimes continues at the same level of severity and frequency. Joanne, the woman who wrote to me describing her twenty years of panic disorder, decided not to have any treatment. Once she found out the true nature of what was happening to her, she realized that since it hadn't gotten any worse in twenty years, it probably never would.

However, in most people the attacks do come at closer intervals and become more severe. Because they seem worse when they happen in public, the sufferer learns to avoid public places. This, of course, sets up the most frequent complication which is agoraphobia. The agoraphobia tends to become more and more restrictive until, like Henrietta, the person becomes housebound.

Treatment for this disease is excellent, and is more often pharmaceutical than psychotherapeutic, although there is a place for both. There are several groups of drugs that work well and are relatively safe. Relief can be expected soon, although treatment may need to be on a long-term basis, often many months. Treatment after agoraphobia begins is still excellent, but relief will probably come slower than before this complication. As in generalized anxiety disorder, depression is another frequent complication.

Obsessive-Compulsive Disorder

The diagnosis of this disease is fairly simple. Whether or not a minor compulsion like lining up three colored pens before working represents an idiosyncracy or a disorder, depends on its effects. Generally, if you spend more than an hour a day at it, it is considered a compulsion rather than a personality quirk. Until recently treatment was through psychotherapy, a long and difficult process that was often not very successful. Today, however, there are several new drugs that offer an entirely different approach and new hope.

Without treatment, obsessive-compulsive disorder may continue at the same level, or may grow even more smothering, as it apparently did for Howard Hughes.

His loss was a tragic loss for us all, perhaps especially tragic, because it may have been due to a disease that could now be treated successfully.

Posttraumatic Stress Disorder

You can recognize the beginnings of this disease if you are continually reliving a horrendous experience. Admitting the need for help is much more difficult. Even the urging of friends and family may not be enough, because of the sufferer's need to block out anything about the experience.

Anyone with this disorder needs professional help urgently. Generally this includes some form of intensive counseling and perhaps short-term medications.

Without professional help the disorder may eventually clear, as it did for David. However, without treatment there often are deep personality scars. If the trauma was inflicted by a person or persons, instead of nature, there may be bitterness, resentment against society, and vindictiveness. While David shows no trace of vindictiveness, he does harbor a deep mistrust of authority and will not even vote.

Treatment, especially early in the disease process, offers early easing of the pain, a quicker return to inner peace, and less likelihood of personality scarring.

Phobias

Phobias are easy to diagnose. Everybody knows someone with a phobia or has unreasonable fears himself and recognizes them as unreasonable. Whether you wish to consider that fear is a disorder or just a personality quirk doesn't really matter. The only critical question is, "Does this interfere with my life? How much do I want to get rid of it?"

Simple phobias are specific—snakes, tunnels, elevators—and can be avoided if you are willing to accept the restrictions. I have a friend with a phobia of closed spaces, especially elevators. He works and lives in a tenth floor apartment in New York City. He has learned that he can tolerate the elevator if he is not alone and it is not crowded. By timing his trips, getting off and on several times on the way up and down if there are too many or too few people, and with some walking, he has managed very well for more than twenty years.

My patient Elwood, who had a tunnel phobia, was willing to accept the restrictions, even job loss. However, after his children complained that they never saw the ocean, he did seek help.

The treatment of simple phobias is usually more behavioral than medical. Social phobias, the fear of doing something embarrassing in public, are more complex, and generally require a combination of medication and psychotherapy.

Depression is a common complication in both simple and social phobias, especially if the phobias become increasingly restrictive.

Without treatment the possible complications of all the anxiety diseases are very real and are statistically measurable. The unmeasured complications, however, may be much worse. These include the results of hasty decisions made when anxious, opportunities ignored when depressed, relationships destroyed when angry, and poor judgments made when preoccupied by worries.

Anxiety disease is worth treating. Treatment works.

WHERE TO GO FOR HELP?

You've decided to ask for help. Where do you start? Usually, as with most ailments, it is best to start with a generalist, a primary care physician.

The medical profession in this country is based on a specialty system. In each specialty there are a series of requirements, prescribed training, and examinations, that qualify a physician to be board certified.

There are three broad specialties, available to people with almost any health problem, and more than two dozen narrow specialties. The narrow specialties restrict their services to people with particular diseases (allergy, oncology), to a specific organ system (cardiology, hematology, psychiatry), or to particular forms of diagnosis or treatment (radiology, surgery). Physicians in any of these fields may be graduates from either a medical or osteopathic college.

The two broad specialties for adults are family medicine and general internal medicine. To be board certified in either requires three years of residency training after graduation from medical or osteopathic school, and passing a series of examinations.

The specialty of family medicine has additional requirements. To remain board certified, its members must have one hundred and fifty hours of continuing education every three years, and pass qualifying examinations every seven years. Residency training in both these fields should prepare graduates for both the diagnosis and treatment of most anxiety disorders. These specialties, together with general pediatrics, are known as the primary care disciplines.

There is another group of primary care physicians known as general practitioners. These are physicians who have not taken the additional training or examinations to become board certified in either internal medicine or family medicine. Some of these physicians have, however, had extra training and experience in the diagnosis and treatment of anxiety disorders. The most basic skill for all physicians is to know the extent and limitations of their own competence. If your physician is a general practitioner, ask about his or her approach to the diagnosis and treatment of anxiety disorders.

Begin with your primary care physician—unless you are certain of the diagnosis, like a toothache or cataract. Most diagnoses, however, are not so certain. Suppose you have a backache. You may decide to go directly to an orthopedic surgeon. However, an orthopedist is only qualified to diagnose and treat problems in the musculoskeletal system. Most backaches are not caused by problems in this system, but are due to a host of other disorders such as bowel problems, menstrual difficulties, tension, shingles, depression, and many more.

Because anxiety disorders cause many physical symptoms, people can find themselves ricocheting from one medical specialty to another looking for THE ANSWER. My businesswoman friend, Edith, saw sixteen physicians in nine or ten specialties within two years. Almost as soon as she completed the studies in one field, her symptoms moved to another. As so often happens, minor abnormalities were discovered and treated vigorously in the hope of helping her. Unfortunately, this treatment resulted in additional complicating side effects such as a bowel inflammation from antibiotics she probably didn't need.

Good health care ought to be coordinated. Every doctor treating a patient should know what every other doctor is doing. It is best for you to have one individual serve this role, one person to be your personal representative, advocate, and interpreter, someone who learns to know you as a whole person. Most often, but not necessarily, this is a primary care physician.

When you decide to seek professional help for your anxiety symptoms, I strongly urge you to start with a primary care practitioner. This is because primary care physicians have a natural role as care coordinators. They also have broad training and experience, and can handle multiple kinds of problems at the same time.

Counselors have training and experience in the various nonpharmacological treatments of anxiety disease. But in most anxiety diseases, people need both drug and nondrug therapy. Knowing this, counselors often team up with physicians so that their patients can have the benefit of both therapies. Many physicians do not have adequate training or skills in psychotherapy and work closely with psychologists, social workers, and other counselors to provide that dimension.

Psychiatrists are physicians with special training and board certification in the diagnosis and treatment of diseases affecting the mind. Most psychiatrists, but not all, have the skills and training to provide both pharmacotherapy and psychotherapy. Patients may go directly to a psychiatrist, but are usually referred by a primary care physician or a counselor.

In addition to these professionals, there are other forms of help available. Most large communities have mental health clinics, staffed by a variety of professionals. In some areas there are also phobia clinics and phobia self-help groups. These can be found through the classified section of the telephone book or through your primary care physician.

What If I Already Have a Personal Physician?

If you have a physician whom you trust, begin there. Ask whether your doctor treats people with anxiety diseases or refers them. If the latter, ask to whom? One of the major advantages in having your own primary care physician is that you have someone who will be able to coordinate your care even if you need to see other professionals. To do this, your doctor needs to know about any health problem you are having and any other health professional you consult. Your doctor may be able to help by making specific recommendations.

How Do I Choose a Physician?

In many parts of the country there are now enough physicians to create a bit of competition. Physicians and psychologists advertise, at least in the yellow pages. You can now be as selective as you wish.

Finding the right doctor for you is an important decision, but not an easy one. The information you need will not be in the advertisement. Nor is there a "User's Guide to Primary Care Physicians in Your Area," but perhaps there should be.

Lacking that, there are several ways to get the information you need:

The first is to ask for a recommendation from someone whose judgment you respect—friends, rabbi or cleric, another physician or dentist. You would like to know if the physician has experience in treating your kind of problem. If the person who is making the recommendation doesn't know, there are other ways to find out.

Next, you need to know the physician's credentials. You need to know the field of practice, whether the doctor is a medical or osteopathic physician if you have a preference, and whether or not the doctor is board certified. The classified section of the telephone directory will usually give you the answers to the first two questions, but not the certification.

If you find a printed announcement or other description, look for the initials after the name. ABIM is for the American Board of Internal Medicine and ABFP is for the American Board of Family Practice.

There are two other sets of initials in use in family medicine that provide useful information, but are not the same. "Member AAFP" means active membership in the American Academy of Family Physicians. "FAAFP" means Fellow of the American Academy of Family Physicians. These designations indicate more than just having paid dues. To continue membership in the Academy, each physician must complete one hundred and fifty hours of continuing medical education every three years. Fellowship is an honor that may be awarded to those who have continued their membership for a long period of time. Most people who are board certified in family medicine, and many general practitioners, have one or both of these added qualifications.

Another way to get credentials is by calling the local medical society or local chapter of the American Academy of Family Physicians. You can also call the American Board of Medical Specialties to check on a specific doctor. The number is (800) 776-2378. You can, of course, call the physician's office, which is now a very common practice. If the answer is that the doctor is "certified," "registered," "board qualified," or any other term except "board certified" in family medicine or internal medicine, it probably means that the doctor is not board certified.

The basic credentials for psychiatrists are certification by the American Board of Psychiatry and Neurology. However, many psychiatrists also have a subspecialty, which might make them either more or less qualified for handling your particular problem. The answer to that question is easy to get; just call the psychiatrist's office and ask.

Credentialing in other fields is not so simple. Many practitioners have a doctorate in psychology; other excellent practitioners have masters' degrees in that or related fields, such as social work. State licensing laws, while fairly uniform for physicians, differ widely for psychologists. Your best source is through a referral from another professional.

You now have some recommended names and you know about their credentials. While that is important, it is not the critical information. Not all primary care physicians are prepared to help you with an anxiety disease. For example, the treatment of a sore throat is pretty standardized; listen, examine, test for strep, and prescribe. Not so with anxiety disease. The understanding of these disorders is changing so rapidly, the means of treatment are so diverse, and the skills to treat so different, that some primary care physicians are not qualified to give you optimum care. How can you tell?

One of my patients is a lesbian woman named Anne, who is a highly educated communications specialist working for a large corporation. She told me about her treatment problems when she first developed panic disorder while living in another city. Anne thought she knew what was happening to her and went to see her primary care physician. The doctor explained that she did not treat anxiety diseases herself, and referred Anne to an excellent psychologist. Anne soon found that the psychologist didn't use medications, which Anne thought she would probably need. Undaunted, Anne then obtained a copy of *Diagnosis and Treatment of Anxiety Disorders: A Physician's Handbook* and gave it to her physician. On the basis of this, the physician agreed to prescribe, the psychologist agreed to continue counseling, and Anne recovered rapidly.

This worked for her, but not everyone has the knowledge, ability, or effrontery to make it happen.

A better way to find out if the doctor can help you is to call the physician's office or ask a friend to call for you if you are having anxiety symptoms. After you have checked credentials there are two questions you should ask:

1. Does the physician treat people with panic attacks? (If you say anxiety disorder, the receptionist might think you are talking about ordinary nervousness.) If you think you might have posttraumatic stress disorder, obsessive-compulsive disorder, or a phobia, you could ask about those specifically instead.
   If the answer is "no," ask to whom the doctor usually refers such patients. (Add the name to your list of possibilities.)
   If the answer is "I don't know," ask to speak to the doctor. If the doctor doesn't understand, say good-bye.
   If the answer is "yes," ask the second question.
2. Does the physician use medication or counseling or both?
   If medication only, ask to whom the doctor refers for counseling.

If answer is unknown, say good-bye.
If there is a regular working relationship with a counselor, make
an appointment with the physician.
If the physician believes in counseling only and not medication,
say good-bye.
If both, make an appointment.

The final way to get the information you need is to make an
appointment to meet with the physician whom you are considering. If
you make the appointment with the understanding that it is just to
become acquainted, most physicians will not charge you.

Tell the doctor that you have been reading this book and that you
think you might have an anxiety disorder. Then ask the same questions
as above.

It is always better to meet your prospective physician before a
crisis. It may not be essential to have a good rapport with your
cardiologist or your neurosurgeon, but it is critical in primary care. You
want to feel entirely comfortable with this person; you want to be able to
confide your most intimate feelings; and you want someone who will
come to care about you as a person. Meeting a person face to face
provides an opportunity to get that "gut feeling" most of us rely on
when deciding whether we could feel close to this person or not.

This was how Anne selected her primary care physician, and the
understanding and candor between them allowed Anne to persuade
her physician to change her treatment policy.

Acquaintance visits have become commonplace in everyday practice and most physicians welcome them. We, too, like to meet the
people we are going to serve before there is a crisis. It helps us
understand you and gives us a chance to begin building the bond
that we both need to rely on in trying to keep you well or help you
manage your health care problems.

What Should You Expect from Your Doctor?

First, you have a right to expect availability. You should not need to wait
long for your first appointment and there should be times available for
your follow-up visits. You should be able to reach your primary care
physician, night or day, if you have a question, as we all expect with
anxiety disease. Or if your doctor is not available, there should be a
good back-up system, someone you can call if needed, such as another

physician or physician assistant who has access to your records. Nothing can be more frightening to a person with anxiety disease who is just beginning treatment, than to be told to call back in two or three days. You need to know that your doctor, perhaps the only person in the world who seems to understand your problem, is available to you.

The second basic requisite is competence. Usually this is demonstrated by taking a careful history, giving a thorough examination, ordering appropriate tests, and avoiding unnecessary tests. The physician should demonstrate an understanding of anxiety disease. You should also expect your physician to take a comprehensive view, considering all of the possibilities, including the possibility that you might be wrong about having an anxiety disease.

You also have a right to expect your primary care physician to learn to know you well and to care about you as a person. One of the ways that caring is demonstrated is by listening; your doctor should be a good listener.

The final characteristic you have a right to expect is that your doctor will be willing to discuss any aspect of your illness—the diagnosis, the recommended treatment and the fee. And you have every right to expect this in your language, not medicalese. DO NOT ACCEPT, "There is a statistical demonstration that this medicament, in prescribed dosage, will diminish symptomatology in a preponderance of cases of this severity," when what really is meant is, "Take the damn pills." DO NOT ACCEPT, "There is a significant element of cardiac pathology masked by the functional overlay of your anxiety," instead of, "You've also got a bad heart."

Ask questions—any questions. As we learned early in medical school, there are no stupid questions; it is only we who are stupid if we fail to ask. No question that is meaningful to you is too trivial to ask. I used to get frequent calls, three or four times a week, from a man named Edward. He was a school teacher of retirement age who lived in a small room downtown. He had a generalized anxiety disorder. For a time his major worry was his bowel movements. He would call me whenever he noted any change in color, size, frequency, or odor. He also documented these findings with a carefully written record. These concerns were genuine. Until he got past this aspect of his anxiety disease, after some months, these were just as traumatic to him as a closet full of boogums and snorklewackers to Binkley or a loose tiger to me. No one but you can know what is crucial or traumatic to you.

Be sure to ask about the side effects of the treatment, whether drugs or psychotherapy, and the possible effects of no treatment, which is a question that is often overlooked.

You have a right to expect much from your physician; your physician also has a right to have some expectations of you.

What Do I as Your Primary Care Doctor Expect from You?

First, I expect you to be completely honest—frank, candid, open, no matter how bizzarre you might think your symptoms sound or how guilty you might feel. I will never laugh at you. I will never accuse you.

Truth is a fundamental expectation in a patient–doctor relationship, but there are exceptions:

I know you may not be totally honest with me until you have learned to know me, to know you can trust me, and to have confidence in me.

I also know that people with addictive diseases or personality disorders cannot be entirely truthful. Dissembling is actually one of the most frequent symptoms of these two disorders. Hilda, the woman with the vodka habit, was honest, but misleading, when she looked me in the eye and solemnly insisted she had only one or two drinks a day, but didn't add that they were six ounces each.

The second expectation is that you will develop confidence. This does not mean a blind belief that I:

Have all the answers.
Always know what will happen next.
Or am always right.

Rather, it means that you will feel sure that I:

Am fully competent in the care that I provide.
Know the extent of my abilities and will get help when needed.
And sincerely care about you as a person and will do all I can to help.

I believe very staunchly that if you cannot develop confidence in me or that I find I cannot trust you, we should find someone else to help you. Truth and confidence are the basic essentials for any successful patient–doctor relationship.

Other Suggestions for the Care and Feeding
of the "Doctus Familius"

You want a physician who will learn to know and care about you as a person, almost by definition a creature with some sensitivity of its own. An indication of your appreciation is always welcome, whether it is in the form of appointments kept, bills paid (or an apology if not), or a simple, "Thanks, doc."

Also appreciated, and a demonstration of some confidence, is an effort either to follow the advice given or to explain why you didn't— "It was too hard," "I forgot," or "I don't think it will help anyway."

The idea of writing this book occurred as I was seeing Ruth on a weekly basis and realized I needed to say the same things over and over again. Ruth is an intelligent woman who paid close attention and had a high degree of confidence. However, her anxiety interfered with her memory, raising continuous doubts and worries. She might benefit, I thought, from being able to read about some of these points between visits.

If this book is to be most helpful to you, your doctor needs to know what you are reading, and what your level of understanding is about anxiety disease. You can assist by urging your doctor to review this or a similar book. In this book your doctor might want to review the chapter summaries, which are designed for your physician's benefit as a quick review of what you have been learning.

SUMMARY

When we have symptoms there are questions we can ask to help us decide if we need treatment:

- Could this symptom be dangerous if not treated? What might happen?
- Does it seem to be getting better or worse, more or less often?
- Does this seem like anything else I've heard about or know about?
- How can I get relief? Does this interfere with my life as I want to live it?
- What does someone else think?

Because each of the six anxiety diseases has a distinct course with different complications, it is important to know when to ignore symptoms and when to go for help.

If you decide to seek treatment, the best place to start is with your primary care physician.

If you need to find a primary care physician, start with recommendations from people you know.

You will need to find out the credentials of the doctor you are considering. Be sure to ask if the doctor treats your kind of problem. If so, ask what kind of treatment is used. Before you decide, make an acquaintance appointment to meet with the doctor.

You have a right to expect availability, competence, and understanding, which means your doctor should be a good listener. Your primary care physician should get to know you well in order to coordinate your health care.

Ask questions; no question is stupid or trivial.

Treat your primary care physician with honesty and openness to develop a good patient–doctor relationship.

Whatever will help the patient get well, I'm in favor of, whether Osteopathy, New Thought, Hindu Yoga, or Christian Science. We need catholicity of mind in the treatment of nervous disorders. We must treat the soul as well as the body.

Frederick Peterson, 1859–1938
(American Poet)

Chapter 12

Help without Medication

You have a diagnosis, you've decided that you need treatment, and you know where to go for help. The next question you're probably asking yourself is, "What is treatment like?" You want to know what is involved in the process, the expected results, the costs, and the hazards. Most people have several major common concerns about treatment.

The first concern of anyone with an anxiety disorder is the all pervasive fear of having another anxiety attack. Anxiety disorders are diseases of fear. Roberta, the woman who feared doctors, would have problems seeking treatment. Henrietta, with agoraphobia, could not possibly go to a physician's office. If you have a social phobia, you will be concerned about who will be watching you in the waiting room or the examining room. With a simple phobia you might be worried about transportation or the small confines of an examining room. If you have panic attacks, you may suffer severe anticipatory anxiety and be anxious about having an attack in a public place.

These concerns are real and may be extremely restrictive, preventing you from getting the help you need. If so, discuss them openly with your family doctor, either by telephone, or if it is easier for you, by letter. If your physician cannot or will not accommodate you, you need to find a different physician.

You will wonder about the nature of the treatment itself. Will I need to stretch out on the couch and talk about my childhood, my sex life, my dreams? Must I be part of a group? Will I have to take drugs that affect my mind? What if I become addicted, or experience all kinds of weird side effects?

These are all legitimate questions. The answer to any or all of them depends on your illness, your doctor's recommendation, your background, but *most of all*, on your decision. Your doctor can explain the kinds of treatment available and make recommendations, but you *always* have the right to accept or reject them.

Another concern is what will "they" think? "They" could be family, friends, co-workers, or neighbors. If you have posttraumatic stress disorder you probably don't care what "they" think. If you have a social phobia, what "they" think may be the most important consideration of all. The concern for most people is somewhere in the middle. "They" will think I'm just not a strong person, that I haven't tried hard enough, that I haven't learned to think more positively, that I am not devout enough, or that I am inadequate in some other way. "They" may be kind about it, pat you on the head and say sweet words. But if the underlying feeling is patronizing, "they" can become a major reason to avoid treatment.

But if I do get past the "what will people think" problem, how long will all this take? Are we talking in terms of a lifetime of therapy or a few weeks of pills? These are questions that need answers before you can make a decision about whether or not to be treated and what kind of treatment you will accept.

Closely akin to the time involved is the cost. If weekly psychotherapeutic sessions are recommended over a long period, the costs will be high. If medication is recommended, what are the actual costs? How much of my treatment might be covered by my health insurance? We all know too well that some modern medications can be extremely expensive.

You need answers to all of these questions before you make a decision. While balancing this equation, however, you also need to ask about the costs of not having treatment. What will continued anxiety disease do to my productivity and my earning capacity? What are the dangers of complications, both psychological and physical? How will my untreated anxiety affect my family?

It is difficult to make any decisions while suffering from anxiety disease or depression. Whenever possible any significant decisions should be postponed. Since the decision about treatment cannot be postponed, lean on those whom you trust the most. Don't be so unreasonable with yourself that you expect to be able to make a quick and correct decision when you are unwell.

TREATMENT GOALS

Most physicians like to establish some goals for treatment. These can be implicit, based on the conversation and unspoken understanding between patient and doctor; or they can be explicit, in which patient and doctor agree on a set of written objectives.

The primary implicit goal is, "Help me feel better." This is certainly a good first goal and perhaps the only one needed at the beginning of treatment. However, as the initial suffering is controlled, you need to consider additional goals.

One of these might be to remove the cause of your disorder, or at least learn to deal with the cause, if it has been discovered. As we have learned, one of the causative agents for anxiety disease is psychosocial. This implies difficulties within the self and the environment. If you identify basic causes within yourself, you may want counseling that will help you alter your inner self, change your response to stress, or improve your coping skills, self esteem and general attitude. If some of the causes are your environment, perhaps you can change that too. Quit your job and take an early retirement as Paul did; look for a different professional milieu; see a marriage counselor or consider a separation and, if necessary, even a divorce.

A third goal might be maintenance. What can you do in the long-run to stay free of symptoms and not worry about the recurrence of this whole anxiety disease cycle?

These are all essential goals and ones in which you have every right to expect help from your physician.

STRATEGY

At this point let's say that you have received a diagnosis, you've decided to seek treatment, and you have delineated your initial goals. Now it is time to develop a treatment strategy. This, again, involves a series of choices. Be a partner in this process. Don't hide behind, "You're the doctor, you decide," or "Doctor knows best." Information is your most important tool. Most people, even some doctors, know little about the anxiety disorders. They seem mysterious since they affect both the mind and body. You need to know what is happening to you, what to expect, and what is expected of you. You need to know the rationale for choosing a particular treatment program. Ask questions, read all of this book, and read anything else your physician may have available and then discuss your options. Discuss these issues with your doctor and with your family. Above all, be sure that you understand what it is that you are about to do.

The simple truth is, people who do not understand or do not believe in a treatment program will not follow it. Appointments are forgotten and medications are changed arbitrarily. "That seemed like too much," or "I was afraid to take them," or "I thought I was feeling better."

On the other hand, people will do anything that they believe will help. Sometimes the belief alone is helpful as in the placebo effect. The patient feels better because of the belief in the treatment, not because of the scientific treatment itself. This effect is real, it helps and we are all subject to it. Besides, if it works, who cares about the scientific validity?

Soon after I started practice my wife and I began to play bridge every Saturday night with our next door neighbors. One night my neighbor, Don, complained of a severe head cold. I told him I had just the medication he needed and got him a pack of little green pills, an old cold remedy recommended by my predecessor in practice.

The following Saturday night I asked him how the pills worked and he said, reluctantly, that he couldn't take them because they caused him severe cramps. I told him this was impossible and that one of the ingredients in the little green pills was actually used for cramps. Essentially I said it was all in his head. He still had the cold and resolved to try the pills again.

The following Saturday night he noted that I had a severe cold and asked me if I had taken the little green pills. He had taken them again, had no more cramps and his cold was gone. I reluctantly admitted that I had tried the little green pills, but had gotten cramps and couldn't take them! The placebo effect is a powerful agent—it had affected both of us.

The results of treatment can be influenced by what we believe will happen.

The minimum requirements for a good treatment plan are:

• An understanding of what the treatment is expected to do

- A standing appointment with the physician; in the beginning, at least every two weeks
- An arrangement to be able to reach the physician, or a back-up person, at all times

DRUGS OR TALK

The final major decision is whether to begin with pharmacotherapy (drugs), psychotherapy (talk), or both. Various forms of psychotherapy are the mainstay of treatment for phobias, adjustment disorder, and posttraumatic stress disorder. Drugs, on the other hand, are usually the mainstay of the treatment for panic disorder and, perhaps, obsessive-compulsive disorder. Generalized anxiety disorder almost always requires a combination.

A general principle is that if the causes are basically psychosocial, the treatment should begin with some form of talk therapy. If the causes are basically biological, as in panic disorder, drug therapy will be needed. Actually, most people will benefit from both forms of therapy. This is logical. We know that chemical changes in the body can cause emotional changes. We also know that emotions can cause chemical changes in the body.

The strategy of combining medical and psychotherapeutic treatments is not strictly confined to anxiety disease treatment. We all respond better to a combination, no matter what kind of ailment. For example, the person who has a broken leg needs some education about the process, reassurance that the fracture was not caused by a bone cancer, and that some pain is normal. It is also important to find out what caused the fracture. Was the missed step accidental? Or was it the result of too much alcohol or inattention due to anxiety? Or was it a sports injury due to lack of conditioning? Psychosocial factors need to be addressed whether the problem is a broken leg or a banged up psyche.

The choice of initial treatment depends on some basic factors, some dependent on you and some dependent on your physician:

1. Diagnosis. Some anxiety disorders respond better to one form of treatment than another.
2. Your health. This is especially important if you have other health problems, are pregnant, or have problems related to aging.

3. Your attitude toward the treatment. If you have a strong antipathy toward the use of drugs, you need to discuss it before a decision is made.
4. The experience and skills of the physician. Each of us has areas of expertise, forms of treatments that have worked well for us, and groups of drugs with which we are most familiar. All of these weigh heavily in the choice of therapy.
5. Addictive potential. The choice of drugs must be made carefully and monitored closely if you have a history of a tendency toward addiction to medications or alcohol. If you have a family history of addiction, it must be considered, as addictive diseases have a strong genetic component.
6. Cost and time. Other significant elements are the differences in cost between generic and nongeneric drugs, individual and group therapy, flooding and desensitization techniques.

Psychotherapy

Psychotherapy means different things to different people. Broadly defined it means using psychological methods to correct psychological disorders. This can be anything from common sense advice to in-depth psychoanalysis. It could be the simple assurance, "Panic attacks feel like they're fatal, but they're not." Or it could be an attempt to alter your inner self.

Scores of techniques have been devised and tried with varying degrees of success. Many of these techniques have not been studied scientifically. Others have been, but with conflicting results. A few have been found to be uniformly helpful. Because the success of these techniques often depends on the individual therapist, scientific studies of psychotherapy are much more difficult and less reliable than studies of drug treatments.

Based on a continuing literature review, and my own experience, I have come to some conclusions about the place of psychotherapy in the treatment of anxiety disorders.

Some people, especially those with simple phobias or adjustment disorder, need only psychotherapy to recover. This is rarely true for the other anxiety diseases.

With the other anxiety diseases, a few people need only medication. A majority, however, respond better to both psychotherapy and pharmacotherapy.

Therapists who do not prescribe drugs tend to believe that psychotherapy is the best treatment. Physicians who are familiar with drug treatment, but not psychotherapy, tend to believe that drugs are the total answer.

There are many forms of psychotherapy, and each has its advocates, professionals who have found that particular techniques work well for their patients. How can so many psychological methods be useful for the same problems? Which is best?

The common denominator probably is not the technique or style, but the enthusiasm, interest, and commitment of the therapist. I believe that the choice of therapy is not nearly as significant as the choice of a therapist.

Counseling

Counseling is a form of psychotherapy, a kind of common sense approach to present or foreseeable problems. It deals with the past only from a historic or genetic viewpoint, and does not delve into developmental issues of the psyche.

If you were a car, "counseling" would fix the broken parts and provide basic maintenance. In-depth forms of "psychotherapy" might address the basic engineering concepts, climatological conditions, and user behavior. There is a proper place for both.

Counseling is usually offered at the first level by the primary care physician. Additional counseling may be offered later on by others such as a professional counselor, a social worker, a psychologist, or a psychiatrist.

In anxiety disorders, counseling can help you get your life back in order, and help you choose a healthier lifestyle.

Most people are dissatisfied with some area of their lives. You might be unhappy in a relationship. You could be unhappy with yourself, with your coping skills or the way you are living your life. You might have a difficult work situation, or perhaps you are having spiritual or social difficulties.

Counseling can help.

- It can help you identify the problems in your life that you want to fix.
- It can help you determine if there is a relationship between your symptoms and your life problems.
- It can help you decide if you want to do something about them and, if so, what you want to do.
- It can provide specific advice (take the damn pills!).

• It can support you during the changes.

If you identify psychosocial factors in your life that are causing or contributing to your anxiety disease, then removing the cause may help you cure the problem. Even if the problem you want to fix is not related to your anxiety disease, counseling may help you find ways to enjoy life more.

There is much in the way we live our lives that affects our health. Counseling by your family doctor can help you choose and live a healthy lifestyle.

The foods we eat have an impact not only on how we feel, but also on our health. There are short-term effects of how we feel after a meal, such as minor indigestion, or the effects of eating too much or too little sugar. There are also long-term effects. For example, a diet high in saturated fats can raise cholesterol levels, causing clogged arteries. Diet has much to do with how we view our bodies, whether we consider ourselves too fat or too thin. Either influences how we view ourselves and how much we like ourselves.

Sleep, irregular hours, and too little or too much of the wrong kind of exercise are other significant factors in our health. Alcohol, tobacco, and caffeine produce immediate effects, but can also affect our future health. Balance between work and play is necessary, as is our perception of what that balance is.

Usually we don't break down, even with significant excesses or deprivations. Our bodies are built to be tough and adaptable; there are good buffer systems against most chemical changes. As to how we feel, most of these details are of little importance on a day-to-day basis. Their real significance is for our future health—and when we are sick.

With any illness, attention to these variables will help mobilize resistance, improve how we feel, and improve our rate of recovery. With an anxiety disease, or any other disease for which there is not a quick and clear-cut cure, attention to these what-your-mother-always-said details can speed up your recovery. It has been said that the next best thing to a good counselor is a pushy mother.

Psychodynamic Psychotherapy

This is an older form of therapy, based on psychoanalytic theory, which is beneficial under certain circumstances. The theory holds that you may have serious problems, or conflicts, originating in your childhood. These conflicts have been repressed and forced into the unconscious so that you are no longer aware of them. Instead your conscious attention is focused inappropriately on some object, often unrelated, like a thunderstorm or tunnel. Treatment begins by trying to uncover the unconscious problem. Once identified, you are helped to learn a more appropriate way of dealing with it. The repressed conflicts may be deeprooted, making them difficult and time consuming to find. Once recognized, facing such conflicts can be painful.

If the repressed problems are a major cause of the anxiety disorder, this method can resolve and prevent a recurrence of anxiety disease. Psychodynamic psychotherapy is a way to achieve basic personality changes, if that was identified as a goal.

Usually this form of treatment is available only through psychologists or psychiatrists, either in private practice or mental health clinics. The costs are variable, depending on the length of treatment needed. The usual, however, is weekly or biweekly sessions over a period of months. The usual access to this form of treatment is by referral from a primary care physician.

Very often psychodynamic psychotherapy is combined with some form of behavior therapy, designed to improve and shorten the process.

Behavior Therapy

The goal of behavior therapy is to change the way we respond. If the mention of a sabre-toothed tiger makes me tremble and sweat and become incoherent, that does me no good. Behavior therapy can help me save that response until a real tiger shows up in my cave.

The theory is that my inappropriate response is something I learned, perhaps as a child going through the usual fears. If that is true, then it is also possible to unlearn it and learn a more useful reaction.

To unlearn a response, I must, in some way, face the thing I fear. There are many techniques and variations I can use to accomplish this. All involve some kind of exposure to the fearsome object or situation, often using images in place of the real thing. If the imaginary tiger does not shred me, I can learn a better way to deal with a real one.

Desensitization is one frequently recommended method. Together the patient and therapist develop a graduated scale, or hierarchy, of frightening scenes. I might first draw a cat, later add stripes, then color it orange and black, then add the sabre teeth (one at a time). The next step might be a stuffed toy and then a trip to the museum.

While the scale is being developed, I learn a muscle relaxation technique, which I use every time I think of the next frightening step on the scale. As I learn to become comfortable on one step, I go to the next. To graduate with honors I might sidle up to the tiger cage at the zoo.

This technique of gradual exposure and learning to cope is the basis for many self-help programs. Instead of a therapist you may use a book and follow each step.

There are many such books available. Self-help regimens are especially beneficial to people with simple or social phobias. In many communities there are phobia societies where people work through their phobias together and share their experiences. It always helps to know that there are others out there who have the same kinds of troubles.

Flooding is a different method of applying the same principle of exposure and relearning. In this process you deliberately expose yourself to the feared object or situation for a prolonged period of time, which is more than three quarters of an hour. You and your therapist drive back and forth through the tunnel or fondle a family of snakes for forty-five minutes or more. If you do survive, contrary to your expectations, and are not arrested for cruising or unseemly behavior, your senses have become so overwhelmed that you are able to learn a new response. This is not a technique to try by yourself.

Behavior therapy is often the first choice for phobias. Recently there have been some studies reporting successful treatment of panic disorders with variations of these methods. Except in the treatment of phobias, behavior therapy is usually combined with drug treatment.

Cognitive Therapy

This entirely new and different treatment technique is based on the theory that the way we act and how we respond to various situations are reflections of our inner thought processes. Since cringing at a paper tiger makes me look foolish, I want to change that way of acting. To do that I need to change my basic thought patterns. Cognitive therapy is a way of identifying my mixed-up thought processes. Then, in a highly structured series of steps, it helps me rearrange my way of thinking.

The place of this form of therapy in the treatment of anxiety diseases has not yet been established. It seems, however, to be most useful in the treatment of social phobias and performance anxiety. This treatment is usually used in combination with other forms of psychotherapy and medications.

Family Therapy

A major premise of family medicine is that everyone is a part of a family system." Each of us is intimately connected to others—family, mate, significant other, fox-hole buddies, or nursing home residents. Anything that happens to us, whether good or bad, affects them; anything that happens to them affects us.

This is the basis of family therapy. Family therapists point out that every cell in our body is part of a tissue; each tissue is part of an organ; each organ is part of a body system; and the combination is a whole person. Each person is part of a group, a community, a nation, a civilization, a planet, a galaxy, a universe. Think of it as a necklace. If you jiggle one part of it, the whole necklace will move, but the strongest jiggle will be the part closest to the part you moved.

This analogy has several implications for understanding anxiety disease.

If the people who are close to you understand how you feel and what you need to do to recover, they can help. Their support will make them part of the solution instead of part of the problem. If they don't understand, thinking your should "get yourself together," they can hinder your recovery, making you feel much worse.

One of the major purposes of this book is to help your family and friends understand your disease and how it affects you.

Because we are each connected, your suffering affects the others around you. Your anxiety or depression can have a contagious quality, resonating within your family. They also may become worried about you and confused over what is happening. They may think you are right in assuming that you are losing your mind or are about to die. This is another reason to treat your anxiety disease—out of consideration for those who care most about you.

A sick family with disruptive relationships, unhealthy attitudes, and unresolved conflicts can be one of the psychosocial causes of anxiety disease. Hilda, who loved vodka, had a major problem because of Max's chauvinistic attitude toward women. She had never learned to cope with it. It was not until she recovered from her addictive disease and learned to manage her anxiety disorder, that she could confront Max and work out a healthy relationship that was meaningful to both of them.

Family conferences are a useful part of treatment for anxiety disease for many people, but not for all. Polly and Bert, the couple with impotency problems, worked out their problems on their own. Robert's wife Elaine was actively involved in his treatment process. Ruth, on the other hand, never felt any need to include her husband although she kept him informed from week to week.

The extent of family involvement depends, of course, on the wishes of the person with the anxiety disease. Participation can be at almost any level—reading this or another book on anxiety, telephone consultations, personal discussions, family conferences, or family therapy.

If you have an anxiety disorder, think about how you want to involve your family and friends. If you were having heart surgery you would want them to know; the outcome of anxiety disease can be just as dramatic or disastrous. You will need all the support you can muster. And if they're contributing to the problem, family therapy could be helpful in bringing that out in the open.

Other Therapies

There are a group of additional techniques that can be used to help, although they are not likely, by themselves, to be curative. Most of these are designed to decrease the effects of stress. For some people they do wonders; for others, nothing. Unfortunately, there is no way of predicting exactly how one individual will respond, so it is a matter of trial and error. If you have generalized anxiety disorder or posttraumatic stress disorder, or even a prolonged adjustment disorder, I recommend that you choose one of these as a part of your treatment plan.

Meditation

Meditation is a simple exercise that lets you tap into your body's innate ability to relax and refresh itself. The forms we are most familiar with are part of an Eastern tradition known for centuries. Scientific studies have shown that meditation lowers the heart and breathing rate and reduces the metabolic rate. The lactate level in the blood declines sharply. These effects are just the opposite of those produced by tension and anxiety. The result is a profoundly relaxed physical state, while the mind stays sharp and alert.

Meditation has been shown to be an effective technique. After extensive research and testing in the laboratories of Harvard Medical School and Boston's Beth Israel Hospital, Dr. Herbert Benson wrote a book about the process called *The Relaxation Response*. He described it as a natural capability that everyone has. You only need to learn how to use it.

There are many forms of meditation, but whatever form they take, they have a number of elements in common. The first is to find a comfortable position. Sitting usually works best so that you won't fall asleep. It is also useful to find a spot that will be free from interruptions—the boss, children, telephones, or tigers. Next you need something to think about.

One simple method is called breath counting. As you sit quietly, think about your breathing. Simply count to four, one count for each full breath. It works this way. Count "one" as you inhale, then exhale; count "two" as you inhale, then exhale. Count to four and then begin again at "one." Some people find it helpful to fill the space when they exhale with the word "and." Then it would go like this: Inhale "one," exhale "and," inhale "two," exhale "and." Repeat the process for fifteen minutes.

The number four is arbitrary. Some disciplines teach eight, some ten, and some begin at one and count sequentially until the session is over. However, the important part is the counting itself. You don't want to have to think about which number you just counted or which one comes next. You just want to count and think about nothing else.

It sounds easy, and it is. However, our minds have a natural tendency to wander. That's okay. Simply brush aside the stray thoughts and return to the counting. Within a few minutes you will feel your body relax, while your mind stays alert.

Another technique is chanting or the use of a mantra—a word that you say over and over. Some schools of thought teach that the content of the word you use is significant. Transcendental meditation (TM) is based on this technique. To learn TM you will need formal instruction, available in many communities.

Other forms of chanting meditation can be self-taught. Choose a short word, phrase, or sentence, anything that says something positive to you: Allah du, God is One, Peace, Aum, or any combination of syllables that is soothing, or meaningful, or both.

Chant softly, or silently in your head, repeating the words over and over. Simply focus your attention on the chanting. As with breath counting, your mind will wander. That's normal. Just gently return to it.

The important part is that you detach yourself from what is happening. Don't judge your thoughts or the content of the mantra. You are doing this for the results. The goal is not to count your breaths or say words. You are doing an exercise with your mind to relax your body.

Fifteen minutes at least once a day is good for a start. You might want to set a timer so you won't worry about how long to practice. As with any other skill, meditation becomes easier the more you do it. The added benefit of daily meditation is that over time, the effects are cumulative. There are many tapes available that will guide you through the meditation process.

Progressive Muscle Relaxation

Progressive muscle relaxation is easy to learn. Many people use it at the beginning of their meditation period or to help them fall asleep at night. It is especially useful if your anxiety symptoms include painfully tightened muscle groups. Often people use it when they feel tense all over. Such tension is exhausting, and relaxing may help fight the fatigue.

The basic technique is to tighten then relax each part of your body, one muscle group at a time. Find a comfortable position, either sitting or lying on your back with your arms at your sides. Start by taking a deep breath. Hold your breath for a count of five, then exhale forcefully through your mouth. Repeat that step and rest a moment.

Next, focus on one leg. Deliberately tense the muscles in your leg and foot. Hold as tight as you can and hold that tension for five seconds. Then let go. Relax the muscles completely. Rest quietly for a few moments, and pay attention to how your body feels. Repeat the process with the other leg, each hand and arm, the stomach, buttocks, neck, and shoulders until each muscle group has been tensed and relaxed. Be sure you relax for a minute after tightening each group of muscles. When you're finished, rest quietly and enjoy the sense of relaxation.

In addition to relaxing you at the time, progressive muscle relaxation also teaches you how to relax muscles at any time during the day. Whether you're in the kitchen, at your desk, in an airport, or in your cave, take a short time out and go through your routine.

As with any other technique, this one works best if done on a daily basis, for about fifteen minutes each time. There are many commercial tapes available that are very helpful in relaxation.

Yoga and T'ai Chi

Another way to achieve relaxation, and exercise your body at the same time, is through yoga or t'ai chi. Both of these disciplines were developed in other cultures thousands of years ago, yet are still found useful in today's society.

Yoga is a system of thought whose goal is the union of mind, body, and spirit. While there are many forms of yoga, the one we are most familiar with is hatha yoga which teaches harmony through breathing and postures.

T'ai chi is one of the oldest Chinese martial arts, often studied today for its health benefits. It, too, teaches harmony through breathing and postures done in slow motion sequences.

Both these traditions are popular today, and many courses and instructors are available. Both disciplines teach movements that tone and strengthen the body and have the added bonus of producing relaxation. Part of this is due to the stretching nature of the movements and part is due to the mental concentration. When your mind is involved in your body's movement, you feel relaxed.

Body Work

Body work includes a range of hands-on therapies. These therapies provide a sense of physical and emotional well being, which many people find helpful. They are especially useful in reducing tension, relieving headaches, backaches, and improving sleep. There are many forms of body therapies available today that are accessible and inexpensive.

Swedish massage is one of the more common therapies. The body is massaged with a series of strokes using a lubricating oil such as almond or mineral oil. It produces a sense of profound relaxation, relieving stress, increasing blood flow to the massaged muscles, and improving flexibility.

Other therapies that may be useful in anxiety are acupressure and shiatsu. Both therapies use finger or hand pressure applied to points, which correspond to the energy points used in acupuncture. The Chinese have used acupressure for more than 5,000 years as a natural healing art. Shiatsu is the Japanese form of that art. Acupressure is a more specific art, while shiatsu includes gentle massage and manipulation of various body parts. Both can relieve symptoms of anxiety and add to your sense of well being.

As with any other therapy, effectiveness will depend on choosing the right therapist. Ask a friend for a referral. If you can't get a referral, make some phone calls and explain what you want. If the therapist you call can't help you, ask for a referral. Make sure the practitioner is a graduate from one of the accredited schools in the therapy you've chosen.

Biofeedback

We have known for a long time that it is possible to learn to control some of our body functions that are usually controlled automatically. Biofeedback teaches you how to gain some control over those functions using an electronic device. For example, if you want to learn to control your blood pressure, you would be hooked up to a machine that monitors your blood pressure. Whenever the blood pressure begins to go down, a signal is given. By concentrating on how that feels, and learning how to do it at will, you can teach yourself to lower your blood pressure.

It is a slow process, but with good instruction and patience it does work. In anxiety disease it is most helpful in learning to control chronic symptoms such as tension headaches.

Exercise

We all know that regular exercise is an important part of good health maintenance. We need to move our bodies to keep our muscles toned, our circulation moving, our joints flexible, and our hearts conditioned.

Exercise has the added benefit of reducing stress. It is a wonderful outlet for excess tension. It stretches muscles, diverts your attention, and helps assure a relaxed, deep sleep. Any activity that increases your heart rate will do, be it running, swimming, walking or aerobic exercises.

One caution, however; if you have panic disorder the excess lactate produced by the muscles as a waste product during strenuous exercise can precipitate an attack.

Walking is great exercise and is the least strenuous. It's the perfect exercise for the nonathlete, for people with medical problems, and for people who don't like to exercise. You don't need fancy clothes or special equipment other than a comfortable pair of shoes.

You can walk just about anywhere. Just lace up your shoes and go. When you're starting, don't worry about your stride or how fast you're walking. Just go for a twenty minute walk. As with any other exercise, it's good to set up a regular walking time and stick to it. Try to commit to at least four days a week, twenty minutes at a time. This simple exercise will provide some of the same cardiovascular and mental benefits as other more strenuous types of exercise. It won't be long until you have a new spring in your step, walking away from tensions and walking toward a new, wonderful sense of well being.

SUMMARY

It is necessary to set some goals for treatment. The requirements of a good treatment program are:

- An understanding of what the treatment will do
- A standing appointment with the doctor, at the start
- An arrangement to be able to reach your doctor at any time

Nondrug therapies include:

- Counseling. It can help you get your life in order and help you choose a healthy lifestyle.
- Psychodynamic psychotherapy. This therapy will help you uncover unconscious problems and learn appropriate ways of dealing with them.
- Behavior therapy. If you have learned an inappropriate response, you can unlearn it and learn a better one. Desensitization and flooding are techniques used in this therapy.
- Cognitive therapy. This treatment is a way of identifying destructive thought processes and doing away with them.
- Family therapy. Because we are each connected to a group, what happens to us happens to them. Our family can help us get well.

Other Techniques

Meditation is a natural method to relax the body with an exercise you do in your mind.

Progressive muscle relaxation relaxes your muscles and relieves tension.

Yoga and t'ai chi disciplines teach movements to tone and strengthen the body and provide the added bonus of producing a relaxed state.

Body work includes a range of hands-on therapies that provide a sense of physical and emotional well being, which many people find helpful. They are especially useful in reducing stress and relieving headaches and backaches.

Biofeedback uses an electronic device to teach you to control some body functions. It is helpful for chronic symptoms such as tension headaches.

Exercise is part of a healthy lifestyle. It is also recommended for relieving stress.

Many aspects of regaining your health, and of staying healthy, do not require medicine or surgery.

Taking drugs can become a habit; so can
avoiding drugs. Both can be injurious to your
health.

                    Thomas L. Leaman, M.D.

Chapter 13

Medications that Heal

Recently medical science has learned much about the use of medications, or drugs, in the treatment of anxiety disorders. Not so long ago people with anxiety disease were simply given sedatives. Usually barbiturates were prescribed for almost any kind of nervous disorder. These drugs produced a calming effect, often sleepiness, but did not treat the anxiety disease itself. They had the additional hazard of leading to addiction; people needed to use more and more to get the same relief.

The first true anxiolytics—literally, anxiety dissolvers—were discovered in the 1960s. The chemical, or generic, names for the first two were chlordiazepoxide and diazepam, marketed under the trade names Librium and Valium, respectively. At that time no one knew how they worked, just that they did.

Based on experience with these drugs, chemical engineers designed new drugs with special properties. They studied the molecules of these new drugs carefully to see which part was responsible for which action, and then made changes to produce the desired effects. Making slight variations in the molecular structure of a drug changes both its good effects and its bad effects. This is a slow process. When a new drug is formulated, it must be tested, first in animals, and then in people. That too, takes time. The studies must include people of all ages with different diagnoses. This is why some of our best drugs have only become available within the past decade, even though the parent drugs were discovered in the 1960s.

WHY USE DRUGS?

We know that there are other forms of treatment available for anxiety disease. We also know that every medication has dangers and side effects. Why not avoid the risk by avoiding drugs altogether? The rationale is simple:

You are ill.
Nondrug treatment may be ineffective.
Drugs can be hazardous, but so is illness.
Drugs work.

The decision to use a drug, or any other form of treatment, should be based on balancing all of these factors. Even psychotherapy can have negative side effects. I recall counseling one woman who was having trouble with her mother-in-law. Her mother-in-law accused her of having an affair while her husband was off in the military service (which was true). I counseled my patient to begin with an apology to her mother-in-law for offending her. After much encouragement, and with considerable trepidation, she did so. Unfortunately, she chose to do it at a family gathering. The result was an enormous knock-down, drag-out fight!

Here are some guidelines to follow when deciding whether or not to use drugs. You will need additional information from your doctor. Remember, though, doctors only recommend; the final decision is always yours.

- Use medication only if your symptoms are disrupting your life. Joanne, who wrote to me about her twenty years of panic attacks, chose not to use medication. Once she knew what was happening to her, the attacks lost their frightening aspect. She preferred to live with the symptoms rather than use medication.
- Use medication only if you have the kind of anxiety disease that drugs can really help. In phobias and posttraumatic stress disorder, medications play only a supportive role.

- Use medication only if you have no complicating factors. Other medical problems and other medications as well as the heavy use of alcohol can make drug therapy more hazardous than helpful. So can an addictive history or being pregnant.

If you decide to use drugs, there are some things you need to know. If your physician doesn't mention them, be sure to ask. Since you know that you have an anxiety disorder, you realize that you may have trouble concentrating and remembering the specifics. Ask your doctor to jot things down for you or, if you are feeling up to it, take notes.

1. Be sure you know what the medication is supposed to do. What will you feel? When will it start working?
2. What side effects might you notice? If so, what should you do?
3. Are there any special limitations like diet, alcohol, or other drugs?
4. Under what conditions should you use the drug? When you have symptoms or regularly? What time of day? Before or after meals? Should you start with a full dose or begin gradually? When should you stop using it, if ever, and how should you stop? What about the possibility of addiction? Can you get hooked?

ADDICTION

Addiction means getting hooked on a drug, so that ever-increasing doses are needed to produce the same desired effect. The dose cannot be withdrawn or reduced without causing physical symptoms. These might include sweating, shaking, nervousness, nausea, palpitations, or even hallucinations. Addiction also implies drug-seeking behavior, a desperate search for the next dose.

Usually, people only become addicted to drugs that give them a feeling of euphoria, which has a spiral effect. Addicts need to continue increasing the dose to get the same high. Sometimes they will use other substances, which may be cheaper or more available, as a booster. These additives enable them to reduce the dose of narcotic they need.

The three principal characteristics of addictive drugs are reinforcement, dependence, and tolerance.

Reinforcement means using one drug to get more of the effects of another. Antianxiety drugs are sometimes used for this purpose. People who use drugs to get high have found that an antianxiety drug will help them get high faster allowing a smaller dose of the narcotic drug. Since medications are usually cheaper than narcotics, they are sold illegally on the street. The street value of antianxiety drugs is relatively low, however, which seems to indicate that while they are used, they are not highly effective for reinforcement.

Research has shown that people who take most antianxiety medications don't get any extra pleasure from them. (Valium and Tranxene may be exceptions.) An experiment was conducted with a group of people who were given either their own antianxiety drug or a placebo, which looked exactly the same. No one knew which they were taking. When they were asked which pill made them feel better immediately, most preferred the placebo, meaning that they did not get high or experience euphoria from the antianxiety drug. Instead, people take their medication because they know it will help them get over their suffering, not because each pill makes them feel good immediately.

Dependency means either a physical or psychological dependence on medication, so that stopping, or suddenly decreasing the dose, causes symptoms. This can and sometimes does happen with antianxiety drugs, especially if they have been used for a long period of time, such as four months or longer.

Often the withdrawal symptoms are exactly the same as the original anxiety symptoms. These can include nervousness, sweating, palpitations, chills, and flushes. So the question is, are the symptoms due to withdrawal, or are they evidence that it's not time to stop the drug?

That may be an impossible question to answer, but there is a good way around it. If the dose is reduced very gradually over several weeks or months, the medication can usually be stopped comfortably. Some people, however, still find it difficult to stop. Some people also need very long-term medication to maintain control of their anxiety disease.

Tolerance means that you need to take increasingly larger doses of the drug to get the same result. In this respect, antianxiety drugs have an outstanding property. While the side effects usually disappear, almost no tolerance develops to the good effects. When first taking these medications, people will often have an annoying drowsiness. Within a week or two, this normally disappears, even though the dose is increased. When the proper dose is reached to control the anxiety symptoms, it does not need to be increased again. The same dose will work, even though the medication is needed for many months. With some medications, such as painkillers, people tend to take more and more over a period of months. This is rarely the case with antianxiety drugs.

In summary, the situation with our present antianxiety drugs is as follows:

Drug abusers use antianxiety drugs as a booster.

Dependency can develop with long-term use; it can usually be handled by tapering off.

Tolerance to the side effects develops, but, fortunately, not to the antianxiety effects.

Antianxiety drugs rarely, if ever, cause true addiction.

BENZODIAZEPINES

The benzodiazepines (BZDs) are the mainstay of drug treatment for anxiety disorders. Benzodiazepine is the chemical name that describes the structure of a family of compounds. Various members of this family can relax muscles, induce sleep, prevent convulsions, and dissolve anxiety.

Particular BZDs have been developed that will promote one of these effects and do little or none of the others. Valium (diazepam), one of the first BZDs discovered, is still in use for all four functions. However, the newer BZDs have been designed to focus on one particular function. Because of this, smaller doses of the drugs are needed to achieve the desired result.

When any drug is taken by mouth, it must first be absorbed by the body before it can take effect. Different drugs are absorbed in different areas of the ten yards or so of the gastrointestinal tract. Among the drugs there are also differences in how long that takes to occur. This can make a difference in how they act. For example, both Valium (diazepam) and Tranxene (clorazepate) are absorbed rapidly, usually within thirty minutes. This means they will very quickly make a difference in how you feel. However, quick as they are, they are not fast enough to help you through a panic attack, which usually lasts less than thirty minutes.

Drugs also differ in how long they stay active in the body. As soon as a drug enters the body, both the liver and kidneys go to work to get rid of it. If it can't be dumped, they try to change it into a compound that is inactive or one that can be eliminated more easily. Naturally, this takes different lengths of time for different compounds. For example, nitroglycerin, which is used for angina, becomes inactive in less than five minutes; a thyroid compound may last as long as two weeks.

Each of the BZDs also differs in how long it stays active. This can be from five to eighteen hours for the shorter ones, and up to one hundred hours for the longer ones. These times are actually given in terms of half-life, the length of time it takes for half of the drug to become inactive. The choice of a longer- or shorter-acting BZD is important because it affects how they are used and what can be expected from them. Physicians know the advantages and disadvantages in either group and the choice depends on the best match-up with your particular needs.

Longer-acting BZDs have two distinct advantages over the shorter-acting. Missing a dose doesn't matter as much because there is enough of the drug left from the last dose to overlap. (However, you should make it up later.) The other advantage is its staying power when the drug is stopped. When BZDs are stopped abruptly problems can arise. However, when a long-acting drug is stopped after a period of use, enough is stored in the body so that it wears off gradually.

Long-acting BZDs also have several potential disadvantages. While not conclusive, some evidence shows that they may cause more initial side effects such as drowsiness, confusion, or impaired performance than their short-term counterparts. When these side effects do occur, they last longer even when the dose is decreased. The other disadvantage is that they tend to accumulate in the body. It is easier to reach a level of overdose because it can sneak up gradually. This is especially a danger in the elderly or chronically ill, because other symptoms may make overdosage of BZDs harder to recognize.

The big advantage of the short-acting BZDs is that there is no accumulation of the drug in the body. This means it is easier to control the exact dose needed to correct the anxiety problem. Two of the short-lasting drugs, Xanax (alprazolam) and Ativan (lorazepam), require a much smaller dosage than other BZDs. If side effects do occur they usually disappear quickly when the dose is reduced.

However, because there is no build-up in the body, it is important to discontinue the drug gradually, or there may be withdrawal symptoms. Another disadvantage is that they require more frequent doses administered at regular times.

Some of the most commonly used BZDs available are shown in Table 15. These drugs are listed in two groupings, the longer- and the

Table 15.   *Commonly Used Benzodiazepines*

Generic name	Trade name	Usual dosage range[a] (mg/day)
	Longer-lasting	
Prazepam	Centrax®	20–60
Chlordiazepoxide	Librium®	15–100
Clorazepate	Tranxene®	15–60
Diazepam	Valium®	4–40
Halazepam	Paxipam®	40–160
	Shorter-lasting	
Lorazepam	Ativan®	2–6
Oxazepam	Serax®	30–90
Alprazolam	Xanax®	.75–4

[a]Be sure to check with your physician before taking any drugs.

shorter-lasting. The first name given is the chemical name. The names in the second column are some of the trade names that are available. The older drugs are also available in generic form, which usually makes them cheaper. These include diazepam, chlordiazepoxide, and lorazepam. The usual dosage for these drugs is given as a range, because each of us has different needs and reacts to drugs differently.

What to Expect

You begin to feel the beneficial effects of a BZD within the first several days. You feel a bit less anxious, nervous, and apprehensive. The physical symptoms of anxiety such as palpitations, sweating, and trembling, occur less often and are not quite so severe. Panic attacks don't usually cease to occur that quickly, but the anticipatory anxiety, that constant fear of another attack, is diminished.

The dosage is usually increased gradually until the full effects are reached, which may take as long as four weeks.

Side Effects

Drugs are used to produce specific desired effects. For example, aspirin is used to relieve headaches, lessen inflammation in joints, and reduce fever. Every medication can sometimes also cause other, usually undesirable, effects. These are called side effects. The possible side effects of aspirin include dizziness, bleeding, abdominal pain, and a disorder called Reye's syndrome in children. With any medication, it is important to know what side effects are possible and how likely it is that they will occur. Some side effects are predictable and depend on the dosage. Others are not predictable because they depend on how you and the drug get along.

The most frequent and expected side effect of BZDs is drowsiness during the first few days. As many as fifteen percent of the people who take it experience this effect. The drowsiness usually disappears within the first week of medication; however, it may be avoided entirely by beginning with a very small dose and increasing it gradually. The other common side effects are dizziness or confusion, although far fewer people experience these problems.

As with most drugs, other side effects can crop up, which are unpredictable. If you have a new symptom soon after you start any new medication, call your physician and ask about it. You need to know if it could be due to the drug, and if so, whether or not you should change the dose, switch drugs, or stop taking drugs completely.

With many drugs the number and intensity of side effects increases the longer they are used; fortunately, this is not true with BZDs. The predictable side effects usually disappear as the medication is continued. It is rarely necessary to stop taking a BZD because of side effects.

How Long Will I Need to Take My BZD?

This depends on the diagnosis and how your body responds. In adjustment disorder BZDs are an adjunct to the main treatment, which is counseling. In this case, the medication will only be used for a short time, probably a few weeks. Sometimes it is recommended that you only take it on an as-needed basis.

Drugs are also an adjunct in posttraumatic stress disorder. Since they are not the main treatment, they are most often used intermittently for short periods of time, ranging from a few weeks to a few months.

In the more chronic diseases such as generalized anxiety disorder and panic attacks, drugs are the mainstay of treatment and are often required for longer periods of time. This, too, is variable. Some people may need to continue the medication indefinitely to control their symptoms.

How to Stop

If you have been taking a BZD on a regular basis for more than a week or two, and your doctor advises you to stop, it is essential to taper off gradually.

Ruth, the patient with panic disorder, was never enthusiastic about taking any medication, and decided at one point that she had recovered, and abruptly stopped taking her short-acting BZD. Four days later she began feeling nervous and apprehensive. Then she began trembling and had abdominal pains. She was discouraged, saying she felt as bad as she did in the beginning. She resumed her full dose of BZD and all the symptoms disappeared quickly. Eventually she was able to stop by tapering off gradually.

Because taking BZDs can lead to physical dependency, gradual withdrawal is important. As in Ruth's case, sudden withdrawal can cause symptoms similar to the original anxiety symptoms. This makes it difficult to tell if the symptoms are due to withdrawal or to the residual anxiety disease. The solution is to reduce the dose very gradually. A general guideline is to reduce the total dose by one-half tablet every two weeks. If the anxiety disease is still present, the symptoms will return, meaning you still need your BZD.

There is an additional danger for people on high doses of short-acting BZDs for a long time. Abrupt withdrawal in these people can cause seizures. Gradual reduction of dosage can prevent this rare complication.

Since we know that one cause of panic disorder is biological, can we expect the medications to cure the disease or only suppress the symptoms? The full answer is not known. Some people need long-term treatment and others do not. It seems quite likely that in some people a healing effect occurs and their bodies seem to regain control of the neurotransmitter complex.

Special Features

Within the two BZD groups, long-lasting and short-lasting, there are also some individual differences.

Valium (diazepam) and Tranxene (clorazepate) are both absorbed rapidly. This can produce a quicker effect, and may also give a sense of feeling high.

Valium has also muscle-relaxing properties, more than any of the other commonly used BZDs. For this reason it is often the drug of choice when muscle tension is a persistent symptom. Sometimes it is used intravenously to stop convulsions.

Librium (chlordiazepoxide) is widely used in the treatment of alcohol withdrawal. Serax (oxazepam) is also recommended for this purpose.

Xanax (alprazolam) has antidepressant as well as anxiolytic properties. If the depressive symptoms accompanying an anxiety disease are not severe, this may be the only medication needed. If it is not sufficient, it may be necessary to add an antidepressant drug as well (see Table 17).

Conclusions

The finding of the BZDs in the 1960s, the discovery of how they work in the 1970s, and the subsequent development of new BZDs has revolutionized the treatment of anxiety diseases. From what I have seen, they have changed these diseases from miserable ailments I could not treat to diseases that are treatable with the full expectation of a happy outcome. To me the diagnosis of anxiety disease has become a welcome one, like the easily removed speck in the eye, a simple dislocation, or a normal delivery. Treatment can be prompt and effective, and my patients are predictably relieved and pleased.

NON-BZD ANXIOLYTICS (OR, A DIFFERENT DRUG TO DISSOLVE ANXIETY)

There is a new group of drugs that show promise in relieving the symptoms of the chronic anxiety diseases, known as the azaspirodecanediones, too new to have a handy nickname. The first drug available in this country is sold as BuSpar, chemically known as buspirone.

Studies have shown that BuSpar is an effective anxiolytic, although slow to act. It may take up to two weeks to become noticeably effective. Because of this it is especially recommended for chronic, rather than acute anxiety problems.

One of BuSpar's advantages is that so far it does not cause physical dependency (like BZDs sometimes do), nor does it seem to have the potential for either physical or emotional addiction. This means it can be useful in people with addictive problems.

Another advantage is that BuSpar does not interact with the BZDs. Because of that, it can be given at the same time as a BZD. This can be helpful to people who are having trouble withdrawing from their BZD because of dependence. Thus, it may help the tapering off process.

Studies have shown that BuSpar and alcohol can be used at the same time. In one study BuSpar taken with alcohol did not affect performance any more than alcohol taken alone. This is significant for those who drink and also need medication for their anxiety disease.

BuSpar apparently does not cause a high feeling. Evidence of this is its street value, meaning how much drug abusers are willing to pay for it. One survey has shown that it was worth only about a third as much as Valium, and only a penny per dose more than placebos.

Since BuSpar is from a different chemical family than the BZDs, the side effects are also different. Most studies report less sedation than with the BZDs. The most common side effects are dizziness, nausea, headache, nervousness, and lightheadedness. These side effects are usually mild and may be avoided by starting with a very small dose.

The most exciting aspect of this new group of drugs is that they are totally unrelated to any other drugs. We can expect that chemical engineering will develop a whole series of new compounds to treat specific anxiety problems. No one knows yet how these drugs work; when that is figured out, it should answer more questions about the chemistry of anxiety disease itself. Unfortunately, the fact that so little is known about the mechanism of these new drugs means that we do not know, as yet, about any long-term ill effects (see Table 16).

BETA BLOCKERS

Another curious group of drugs used to treat many other diseases can also have a role in managing some social phobias. The name comes from their ability to block the action of certain body chemicals at locations called beta receptors in the autonomic nervous system. This blocking action is effective in many cardiovascular disorders, including high blood pressure, angina pectoris, and migraine.

These drugs are especially useful to combat performance anxiety such as stage fright and examination nerves. They work, as they do

Table 16.   *Other Drugs Used in Anxiety Disease*

Chemical name or group	Trade name[a]	Comments	Usual dosage range[b] (mg/day)
Beta blockers	Inderal®	Useful in performance anxiety	10–40
	Tenormin®	Useful in social phobias	50–100
Buspirone	BuSpar®	Slow to act	15–60
		No dependency	
MAO inhibitor	Nardil®	Severe food restrictions	45–75

[a]In some categories there are many other trade names.
[b]Be sure to check with your physician before taking any drugs.

when given for cardiovascular disorders, by blocking some of the overactivity of the autonomic nervous system. This prevents trembling, palpitations, rapid breathing, sweating, flushing, and related symptoms. One of the most commonly used beta blockers for this purpose is Inderal (propanolol).

Inderal is used by taking a single dose about thirty to forty-five minutes before a performance or presentation. It blocks autonomic symptoms such as rapid pulse and breathing, sweating, lightheadedness, and trembling. Since these symptoms are blocked and the performers know they are blocked, there is a sense of relief that allows them to do their best and enjoy the process.

The only likely side effect for this single-dose therapy might be some sense of fatigue. These drugs are not advised for people who have congestive heart failure, are subject to bronchial asthma, or have an abnormally slow pulse.

Some people have much more generalized social phobias. Instead of fears about a specific event, like public speaking or examinations, they have autonomic symptoms in many different social situations. Since the symptoms are unpredictable, a single, preperformance dose obviously won't work. These people have gotten some relief from beta blockers that are taken once a day on a continuing basis. For this problem, one frequently used beta blocker is Tenormin (atenolol). Although quite infrequent, the principal side effects are dizziness and nausea.

Beta blockers do not erase the social phobia. However, they can make life much more enjoyable while other, nonpharmacological, treatments are being used to overcome the basic disease (see Table 8).

ANTIDEPRESSANTS

This group of drugs, which includes several families, has provided enormous help and hope for people with anxiety disorders. Antidepressants were designed specifically for people with depression; however, most people who have an anxiety disorder also have depressive symptoms during the course of their disease. (Table 17 shows commonly used drugs for treatment of depression accompanying anxiety disease.)

Serendipitously, some of these drugs are also effective for panic disorder.

The first effective antidepressants were available before the BZDs. They were a great breakthrough in the treatment of depression. Before this our only treatment was psychotherapy, which was of limited value, and stimulants such as Ritalin and the amphetamines. These do not really counteract depression, but provide only a short, temporary euphoria.

While some of these drugs have been in use for decades, our understanding of how they work is still incomplete. It is known that they act within the complex neurotransmitter systems. The theory is that depressive symptoms are caused by an excess of certain chemicals, or a deficiency of others that are meant to oppose them.

One fact about antidepressants is certain: they work.

Tricyclic Antidepressants

The tricyclics were the first group of these drugs, so named because of their chemical structure. Each member of this drug family has a similar chemical configuration—three hexagonal rings attached to each other. Their differences depend on the other chemical components attached to these rings. Some of the most common members of this family currently in use are Anafranil (clomipramine), Asendin (amox-

Table 17. *Commonly Used Drugs for Treatment of Depression Accompanying Anxiety Disease*

Chemical name or group	Trade name[a]	Comments	Usual dosage range[b] (mg/day)
Tricyclics	Anafranil®	Obsessive-compulsive disorder	25–200
	Asendin®		75–200
	Aventyl®		25–100
	Elavil®		75–150
	Norpramin®	Also used in panic disorder	75–150
	Pertofrane®	Also used in panic disorder	75–150
	Sinequan®		75–150
	Surmontil®		75–150
	Tofranil®	Also used in panic disorder	75–150
	Vivactil®		15–40
BZD	Xanax®		.75–4
Others	Desyrel®		150–200
	Ludiomil®		75–150
	Prozac®		20
	Wellbutrin®		200

[a]In some categories there are many other trade names.
[b]Be sure to check with your physician before taking any drugs.

apine), Aventyl (nortriptyline), Elavil (amitriptyline), Norpramin (desipramine), Pertofrane (desipramine), Sinequan (doxepin), Surmontil (trimipramine), Tofranil (imipramine), and Vivactil (protriptyline).

As you might surmise from the similar sounding chemical names, many of these drugs are quite like each other, with their molecules altered slightly to change their effects or side effects.

Nontricyclic Antidepressants

There are other antidepressants that are nontricyclic. They differ, not only from the tricyclic family, but also from each other. These include Desyrel (trazodone), Ludiomil (maprotiline), Prozac (fluoxetine), and Wellbutrin (bupropion).

How Used

Antidepressants are started at a low dose to minimize the annoying side effects and to observe the start of any more serious effects. The dose is generally increased over a period of weeks. Because all of these drugs are slow to act, it is usually ten days to two weeks before the person notices improvement. The improvement is also quite gradual. I usually tell patients not to expect any change during the first week. Then during the second week to expect some slight lifting of the load. Things won't seem quite as dark; crying spells may be shorter and come less frequently. There should be a little less of the overwhelming sense of fatigue. After two weeks people usually agree that their lives might not seem quite so hopeless, at least not all of the time. After another two weeks they usually are able to make a positive statement with some confidence. Soon thereafter they are able to manage a real smile, not just a forced baring of the teeth.

Some of the tricyclics, especially Tofranil, Norpramin, and Pertofrane, are used in treating panic disorder. They effectively decrease the frequency and severity of the panic attacks, but they do not decrease the anticipatory anxiety. In fact, sometimes during the first week or so, people may notice an increase in anxiety. If the drug is continued, however, this usually disappears. After the initial phase of treatment, and the frequency and severity of the attacks subside, then both anticipatory anxiety and depression may also respond.

After an effective dose level is reached and the panic attacks are blocked, the same dosage is continued for two months. After this the dose may be gradually reduced to a maintenance level, a fraction of the full treatment dose. If the symptoms come back, the dose is simply increased for a longer period of time. After satisfactory maintenance for some months, the drug may be gradually withdrawn. This works for some people, but not for others. Some people will need to stay on a maintenance dose indefinitely to prevent recurrence of symptoms. This can be done safely and effectively.

When antidepressants are used for the treatment of other anxiety diseases, they are used in a similar manner, but can often be discontinued sooner than in panic disorder. Fortunately, they can be used at the same time as BZDs, although it is not certain that they can be used safely with BuSpar. Antidepressants are started at a low dose, increased gradually to an effective level, maintained for a period (I usually wait until several weeks after patients are sure they don't need it any more), then gradually discontinued.

Side Effects

The unwanted effects of antidepressants can be merely a nuisance or a serious problem. The most common side effects with tricyclics are dilated pupils causing blurred vision, dry mouth, trouble urinating, constipation, or drowsiness. These effects usually disappear with continued use and may sometimes be avoided by starting with a low dose and increasing slowly. Most of these symptoms are manageable. Chewing sugarless gum may help the dry mouth. Milk of magnesia is suggested for constipation. There are drugs that may counteract the urinary retention, but unless the retention is minimal, the antidepressant probably should be stopped.

Less frequent, but more serious side effects, have to do with the heart. Antidepressants may affect both the heart rate and rhythm, and can cause a significant drop in blood pressure.

Tricyclics should be used cautiously in people with a history of heart disease, glaucoma, or urinary retention. They should also be avoided in those with a history of seizure disorder. There have been some reported incidents of such people having convulsions on these drugs.

The side effects of the nontricyclic antidepressants, Desyrel, Ludiomil, and Wellbutrin, are about the same as for the tricyclics.

Prozac (fluoxetine) is one of the most widely prescribed drugs for depression. It has a very different set of side effects. The most frequent, occurring in ten or fifteen percent of the people taking the drug, are nervousness, anxiety, and loss of sleep. This is a serious consideration if you need to take an antidepressant and already have anxiety disease.

The successful treatment of obsessive-compulsive disorder with drugs is quite new and deserves special mention. Anafranil (clomipramine), a tricyclic antidepressant, is specifically recommended for this purpose. Because the drug can cause sedation and has potentially dangerous side effects, including seizures and heart irregularities, it should be prescribed only by someone who is familiar with its use. Several other drugs, including Prozac, are currently being investigated for this use as well.

Large overdoses of the antidepressants are dangerous, and can be fatal. This is a serious concern when they are used by anyone who is not a totally reliable pill taker, or who has any potential for suicide. One precaution is to agree on a family monitor, someone in the family who will be responsible for measuring out the doses.

The manufacturers recommend that antidepressants not be taken with alcohol. It is also important, as with any other drugs, to be sure that there is no conflict between this drug and any other drug that you may need to take.

Even though these medications can be agonizingly slow to work, have aggravating side effects, and come with all kinds of precautions, they truly are wonder drugs. Depression is one of the most miserable feelings humans can experience. The relief antidepressants can give has been described as being like the dawning of a beautiful day after a very long dark night.

MAO INHIBITORS

Another group of drugs with a special role in the treatment of anxiety disorders is called monoamine oxidase inhibitors (MAOs). These drugs function by altering the neurotransmitters in the central nervous system in ways that are not fully understood.

At the present time these drugs are usually reserved for special situations. They are effective antidepressants and excellent for controlling panic disorder. Usually these two diseases respond well to our first-line medications, BZDs and standard antidepressants, combined with psychotherapy. But occasionally, even with full doses after several months, these diseases are not controlled. In that case, the MAOs may prove to be a great boon.

The reason for withholding them and using them as a back-up system is that they have potentially serious side effects and hazards. These drugs have powerful effects on many of the body's own chemicals and interact dangerously with many commonly used medications, such as simple cold remedies, and with many ordinary foods like cheese and wine.

The effects that may occur, even when following the medication and dietary restrictions, are many. In addition to the usual side effects of the tricyclics, the list of symptoms that may occur includes sudden lightheadedness (especially when getting up), gastrointestinal problems, muscle twitches, restlessness, rash, jaundice, and swelling of the hands and feet.

The foods that must be avoided are those that are high in tyramine or tryptophan (not usually listed among the ingredients). There is a long list of such foods but it includes cheese, bananas, avocados, smoked foods, red wine, beer, soy sauce, caffeine, and yogurt. It is possible to eat some of these foods and have no symptoms; however, they may trigger a violent hypertensive crisis. This is a sudden increase in blood pressure, with headache, rapid heart beat, chest pain, sweating, nausea, and vomiting. Emergency care is required and the symptoms can be reversed with prompt treatment.

All of this paints a frightening scene. However, most people who take MAOs, and follow the strictly prescribed dietary and medication lists, experience only minimal, nondangerous side effects. If the first-line drugs have failed to help, most people suffering from either depression or panic attacks are so miserable that they are willing to follow any kind of diet, and even to take some risks. Continuing with these diseases unchecked is also risky. But as stated throughout this book you should take medication only in consultation with a physician who has been well apprised of your condition.

SUMMARY

Modern antianxiety drugs have the following properties:

- Dependency can develop with long-term use; it can be handled by tapering off.
- Tolerance to the side effects develops, but not to the antianxiety effects.
- Antianxiety drugs are rarely addictive.

Benzodiazepines are the mainstay of treatment for anxiety disorders. Members of this drug family can relax muscles, cause sleepiness, prevent convulsions, and dissolve anxiety. Different BZDs will focus on one of these actions and none of the others.

A non-BZD that relieves anxiety is BuSpar (buspirone). While it is slow to act, it does not cause dependency.

Beta blockers belong to a different group of drugs that block some of the overactivity of the autonomic nervous system. They are useful for performance anxiety and social phobias.

Antidepressants were designed for people with depression; however, most people who have an anxiety disorder also have some depressive symptoms during the course of their illness. Some antidepressants are also used in panic disorder. Another antidepressant, Anafranil, is used in obsessive-compulsive disorder.

MAO inhibitors have a special role in the treatment of anxiety disorders. They are effective antidepressants and excellent for controlling panic disorder. Because of possible side effects and hazards, these drugs are only used as a back-up system.

The discovery of safe and effective pharmacological treatment of anxiety disease is one of the answers that heal.

One hug is worth a thousand nags.
Thomas L. Leaman, M.D.

Chapter 14

"There's No Place Like Home"*

John Howard Payne
1791–1852
American Playwright and Actor

Dear Doctor Leaman,

Thank you again for explaining Harry's anxiety disease to me. Once I understood it and talked with Harry, we both felt better.

These past weeks have been hard. Harry has been so irritable and jumpy. When he wasn't yelling at me or the kids all he did was sleep, or complain about how tired he was. I think it was him being so tired all the time that was really getting to me. After all, he never did anything. Why should he be so tired? Then he started in on how my cooking was upsetting his stomach. That really made me mad. My cooking was good enough before.

Then you tell him he's got anxiety disease. Great, I thought. I knew all the time, it was just his nerves. Until you explained it, I didn't understand about anxiety disease being a real disease and all. Now I know he's actually sick and I believe I can help him.

So before he couldn't make up his mind about what to wear. He'd just stare at the closet. So the other night I thought I would help him and left out some clothes for him. When he saw them in the morning, he didn't say much. He just looked at me funny. Then he gave me a big hug.

Now I know we're in this together. Thanks, Doc.

Very truly yours,
Sara

This letter and similar comments from others have helped me understand aspects of anxiety disease that I had never thought about before. Spouses and other family members do not understand anxiety disease any better than the patients who have it. This causes not only a hellish nightmare for them, but has to make the anxiety sufferer feel even worse.

This is one of the reasons I wrote this book. It's not intended only for the person with anxiety disease, but also for Sara and for others like her. Everyone who wants to understand anxiety disease and support those who have it, needs some basic information. If you, as a person with anxiety disease, think you may be going out of your mind, what else should your family think? What could they think when you suddenly leave your grocery cart in the store and run outside? When you keep getting attacks of chest pain and the emergency room doctor says there is nothing wrong? When you won't eat in a restaurant with friends, but prefer to wait in the car?

It is hard for anyone to recover from a paralyzing stroke without loving support. It is just as hard, but should not take as long, with an anxiety disease. This chapter tells how to give that support. If someone you love or care about has an anxiety disease, this chapter will help you create a supporting world for that person.

What can you do to help?

BE SURE OF THE DIAGNOSIS

The first thing to do is to be sure of the diagnosis. Suppose your friend is having symptoms, but has not sought professional help. You want to be sure it is an anxiety disease and not something else.

You can be pretty sure of your diagnosis with simple phobias. The real question is whether or not they cause enough anguish or interfere with life enough to be worth going through treatment.

Adjustment disorder is also easy to recognize if there has been a stressful situation with prolonged anxiety symptoms. However, if there are any physical symptoms, your friend does need to see a doctor. Anxiety disease can cause a variety of intense physical symptoms, but so do many other diseases. Anxiety disease can also trigger many other ailments like peptic ulcer, heart disease, and asthma. Do not make the mistake of assuming that various symptoms are due to anxiety and therefore will not be life threatening.

All of the other forms of anxiety disease need professional help: generalized anxiety disorder, panic attacks, posttraumatic stress disorder, and obsessive-compulsive disorder. So even if you feel sure of your own diagnosis, urge your friend to seek professional help.

When Robert had his first attack of chest pain, Elaine rushed him to the hospital. At first he rejected the diagnosis of anxiety disease, and certainly wouldn't agree to take any drugs. When he continued to get chest pains, he reconsidered, and finally was able to accept the diagnosis. However, if he gets another attack of chest pain sometime and experiences symptoms of sweating and shortness of breath, there is a danger that he will say, "It's only anxiety." It could be a heart attack; procrastination could be fatal. Unfortunately, diseases don't happen on a one-to-a-customer basis. Anxiety disease doesn't keep someone from getting something else. Find out for sure. See a doctor.

Suppose your friend refuses to go for help, even for an initial diagnosis? Try to understand why. The probable reason is fear, which is the basic symptom in all anxiety disorders. Remember Roberta who had an overwhelming fear of all things medical and doctor related. That phobia nearly cost her her life because of untreated diabetes and an untreated abdominal tumor. It took a fractured toe, with enough pain and worry, to force her past the fear to seek medical help.

Understanding some of the causes will help to abate fear, or at least make it more tolerable. Urge your friend to use this book and read the first few chapters, or at least the summaries.

Fear is also more tolerable when we are not alone. Remember how comforting it is to have someone in the house with you when you hear the sounds of a door latch opening, or a footstep upstairs, or when you are lost in an unfamiliar city, or when the airplane suddenly seems to drop. The other person may be a perfect stranger, and no more powerful than you, but there is comfort in having someone there.

So be physically and emotionally available to your friend. Be there physically to go along to the doctor's office or to offer comfort when the symptoms attack. But also, be there emotionally. Your friend needs uncritical, nonjudgmental support. If you cannot genuinely feel uncritical or nonjudgmental, perhaps you should get counseling for yourself, or stay away.

If your friend cannot leave the house to go for help because of agoraphobia, ask the doctor to make a home call. If your doctor doesn't make them, find one who does. Most family physicians do make home calls.

Making certain of the diagnosis is the first step in creating a supportive environment.

HOW TO HELP

The next step is knowing how to be helpful to your friend or loved one. How do you act toward someone with anxiety disease? The simple answer is, don't act. Be natural. Be yourself. It sounds easy, but it isn't.

Anyone who is troubled by personal doubts or is overwhelmed by unnamed fears needs some solid ground, some rock of dependence. To be effective that rock should be someone whose honesty and candor are reliable, whose love and caring are absolute. A person with anxiety disease who does not have that kind of support will feel like a free-floating balloon. If you are to be that anchor, that kind of friend, you cannot waffle in the truth.

Try to be aware of your friend's feelings, but also be honest about your interpretation of those feelings.

- Don't minimize the scary feelings. "It's nothing—everybody has a little fear."
- Don't ignore the feelings. "I know you are afraid of flying, but I got two tickets anyway."
- Don't denigrate your friend. "You wimp, real men like to fly."
- Don't exaggerate the problem. "My god! You have a phobia! Quick! Call 911."

But what if these are your real thoughts? How can you be both honest and helpful? Here are some suggestions of positive things you can do.

First, acknowledge that the problem is real. "I know it really makes you feel miserable, even at the mention of it."

Next, you both need to learn about it. "I don't see any reason for your fear and neither do you, but there must be some kind of explanation. Let's find out about it."

It is almost always a mistake to assume that any one person is the first human to experience a particular feeling. So no matter how unusual your friend's feelings and fears, it is safe to assume that others have had them. In that case, someone must know more about them. You and your friend can learn more about this disease together. Read all the parts in this and other books that have anything to do with your friend.

Find professional help and ask questions—lots of questions. And be sure to let the doctor know what you're reading.

You can offer help. You know that a person with anxiety disease has trouble focusing, trouble concentrating, and trouble making decisions. One of the worst parts of anxiety disease is accepting that these simple tasks of living are suddenly hard to do. So help. Instead of, "What shall we do this evening?" offer specific suggestions: "Let's go see *Superman*," or limited choices, "Do you want to go for a walk or watch TV?" Until your loved one is feeling better, offer to make the decisions and do the bulk of the concentrating and planning.

And whatever you do, punctuate everything with hugs. People need to be touched. That is especially so with people who are ill. Your friend may not know how to ask for it, so reach over and touch. You can say more with a hug or an arm around the shoulders than you ever can with words. Remember, it takes more than one hug a day to keep the snorklewackers at bay.

For many years my wife and I have had a cartoon strip of a small boy and his pet mouse on our kitchen bulletin board. The paper is so old and yellowed, I can no longer read the name of the strip or the cartoonist. The first two frames show the boy picking up his mouse friend and giving it an affectionate hug. The last two frames show a very happy mouse saying, "It's a scientific fact. A hug contains minimum daily requirements for everything you need."

Be willing to discuss anything openly. Perhaps your friend has decided to let the small anxieties live in the closet. That's okay, but your friend may still want to talk about them sometimes. That is easier if you both acknowledge their existence. Mr. T. Bailey Elkins had an adjustment disorder because of his fear over losing the big money deal. He needed to share that fear with his wife. When it was out of the closet and they discussed it openly, Mr. Elkins was well on his way to recovery.

The next step in supporting your friend is to learn empathy, not just sympathy. Sympathy means feeling sorry for someone. Empathy is feeling what the other person feels. It also means letting your friend know that you share those feelings. "I hate feeling frightened. It must be worse for you to feel that way even when you know the danger is not as bad as it feels."

To be empathetic you must learn to be an active listener. Most of the time we are surrounded by the sounds of talk, TV, radio, machinery, nature, and our own sounds. From all of this cacophony we sort out what we want to hear while ignoring the rest, unless there is something that suddenly grabs our attention like a shriek, the song of an unknown bird, or the mention of our name.

Such passive listening is how most of us listen during the day. In a conversation we pause at intervals to make sure others are hearing us. After a grunt, nod, or comment, we go on, thinking we have the other's undivided attention. That might not be true, however. The other person's mind may be elsewhere and the response simply automatic.

When your friend wants to confide innermost feelings, this demands your absolute, focused attention. "I feel like I'm going to die," warrants more than a nonchalant, "Oh? I'm sorry to hear that."

Active listening means deliberately focusing your complete attention on another person and what that person is saying. This requires blocking out all other sounds and distractions and ceasing all other activities. It amounts to saying, "What you have to say is more important to me at this moment than anything else."

To listen actively also means that you let the other person know you are totally attentive. You can do this with eye contact and with body language when you sit close, leaning toward the other person with your arms uncrossed and your hands at rest. You can also do it with reflection, which is a way of answering nonjudgmentally to let the other person know you heard exactly what was said. For example, your friend says:

> "Your meatballs upset my stomach."
> "You feel nauseous?" you answer, letting your friend know you heard.
> "Yes, and my stomach hurts."
> "I'm sorry you feel so badly. Do you want to take something for it?"

Listening actively does not mean defending yourself with, "They didn't bother anybody else."

Nor does it mean ignoring the other's comments by responding, "Mother is coming for the weekend." Active listening is a way of letting your friend know you heard and understood. You let your friend know that you are concerned and that you are not sitting in judgment.

HOME SWEET HOME

The concept of home conjures up comforting thoughts of security and understanding, perhaps even hugging and being hugged. Home plate in baseball is the starting point, and the place of victorious return. Home in parcheesi is the goal of the game, a place of security.

In the best sense of the word, home is more than a haven and a place of appreciation. It is also a place of nurture, growth, and encouragement.

Humans are social creatures and prefer living in families or groups, for security:

Make fire, keep tiger out of cave.

and encouragement:

Take club, get mate.

and nurture:

Eat meat, get strong.

As Sara described in her letter, understanding more about her husband's disease helped her assume a new role. Instead of being accusatory, she became consoling and supportive. She learned to substitute hugging for nagging. Her husband, instead of needing to defend himself, felt encouraged.

People with anxiety disease need a home, a place that encompasses all of the nurturing meanings of home. They need a home that is safe from outside attack, misunderstanding, and stress. They need a home to recoup, to grow, and to feel the support of a family.

Frank and Francine were a study in contrasts. Francine was an exuberant person who loved sports and parties, almost any activity, as long as it included a crowd. Frank on the other hand, was quiet, retiring, and sensitive, and detested crowds.

They had married as soon as they finished college. Francine worked as a receptionist and Frank specialized in tax work as an assistant to a CPA. Despite their differences, their marriage seemed solid. They were both happy when Francine became pregnant, although Frank was worried. He worried because Francine insisted on continuing her daily two-mile run. He worried about whether or not the baby would be okay; he also worried about how they were going to save enough for the child's college education. He seemed to have an unlimited supply of worries.

Francine charged into motherhood with unbounded enthusiasm. She read everything available, trying and buying everything anyone recommended. She soon announced that she was determined to have four more—"At least a basketball team." Frank's only comment was, "We'll see."

Their marriage went along well until what Frank later described as "that damn trip to Washington." Francine had always wanted to go to Washington to see the cherry blossoms. Until then they had spent vacation time camping at state parks, which they both loved. Frank finally agreed to the trip, and all went well until they got to the Washington Monument. Francine wanted to climb the steps, but Frank refused. Francine then wanted to take the elevator to the top, but Frank tried to convince her that the line was too long and they didn't have time to wait. But the line was short and moved quickly. Finally, he had to confess his carefully protected secret. He was afraid of heights; he could not go up the elevator.

Francine thought that this was absolutely hilarious. She laughed at him. She "made a big fuss right in front of that whole crowd." Francine thought they should go up anyway so he would "get over it." Frank really wanted to show her that he could, but he simply could not do it. Even the thought of it made him feel panicky. He tried to hide his symptoms from Francine and hurried her off to the Lincoln Memorial.

Always ashamed of his fear, Frank did not even call it a phobia. He had carefully planned his life to avoid heights and especially to avoid telling Francine. As he had suspected, now that the secret was out, things got worse. Francine did not want to discuss the problem, but she was delighted to tell their friends about their trip to Washington—*all* about it.

Then Frank began getting other symptoms. The first was an attack of abdominal pain. It looked like the onset of appendicitis, but the pain disappeared even before all the tests were completed. Then, over several months, he had attacks of severe headaches, followed by more abdominal pain. He also had joint pains, occasionally requiring the use of a cane. For the first time his blood pressure became elevated. He then had two episodes of sudden shortness of breath complicated by palpitations. I believed that all of those symptoms, and possibly the elevated blood pressure, were a direct product of his anxiety disorder. But Frank refused to accept my interpretation.

With each new episode, Francine became extremely solicitous, even tender. At first she embraced her new role of nurse with the same enthusiasm she did everything else. Frank suffered bravely.

Over time, however, Frank and Francine drifted apart. Though they continued to live together, their lives became separate. Francine became absorbed with their teenager and her latest passion, tennis.

The story as I heard it was strictly from Frank's viewpoint. Francine has never agreed to a family conference, or rather when she has agreed, she always had to cancel for some reason. Over the years she has become less tolerant of Frank's multiple symptoms, and is at times derisive. "You have to expect some aches and pains. You're almost 40 and you don't exercise." However, when the symptoms seem serious, like a trip to the emergency room for chest pains, she resumes her nurse role.

Frank has continued to fear heights, but the topic is never mentioned at home. All family travel has been planned to avoid high places. Frank has had two offers of advancement but turned them down. Both would have required him to work in high-rise buildings, which by his definition is over three stories. He could not do it, and he never mentioned these offers to Francine.

Twice I persuaded him to see a psychiatrist for help. The first time, Francine became so incensed at the cost that Frank cancelled after two appointments. I then persuaded a psychiatrist friend to see Frank at a reduced fee. Frank kept five or six appointments and thought that he might be getting better. He had even ventured to the third floor of the local department store by himself. But Francine said that at that rate of progress she'd be in a nursing home and wouldn't care by the time he was able to fly to Hawaii, her lifelong dream. Frank cancelled further appointments.

Frank is a hurt and unhappy man. Although he won't admit it, he has become comfortable with his ill health, and his repeated episodes of seemingly unrelated symptoms. He simply cannot see the relationship between his personal and physical problems. He needs his symptoms; they are an excuse for his limitations. He has little insight into his basic illness and is still ashamed of his phobia.

Frank has never found a home. He has never found a place where he could be comfortable and get the attention he craves without the need for symptoms. He needs a place where he can be himself without becoming the butt of laughter. Ridicule hurts, but when it comes from friends or loved ones it wounds deeper. Apparently, Frank never recovered from his wounds on "that damn trip to Washington."

Frank needs understanding to help him face his anxiety disease and recognize it for what it is—a disease, not a character flaw for which he should feel ashamed. Frank and Francine both need to recognize this disease for what it is—a family problem—and make decisions that are good for both of them. It might be foregoing the new car and investing whatever money and time it takes to get well. Or perhaps they would decide to go their separate ways. Frank remains an unhappy, and perhaps because of this, an unhealthy man, unwilling to continue therapy without Francine's support. I can't really tell whether Francine is happy or not. She is not willing to discuss anything so "heavy." And as their doctor I am not happy either, with my inability to change their self-destructive course.

Contrast this sad story with those of some other people. Ruth was never uncomfortable at home. Her husband was always supportive during the long period of her increasing symptoms. He was attentive to her troubles and tried to help in any way he could. He went shopping, ran errands, and, as a last full measure of devotion, offered to attend the PTA meetings. He didn't understand her symptoms anymore than she did, but he never doubted they were real. He encouraged her frequent and expensive medical visits. When the diagnosis was finally made, he accepted it. He was able to understand and accept Ruth's explanation of what she was learning. As usual, I suggested a family conference, but neither of them felt the need. Ruth always knew she had a safe place, a home where she was accepted, appreciated, staunchly supported, and loved.

Robert's panic disorder seemed to begin abruptly with an attack of chest pain. During this and a subsequent episode, Elaine shared his fear of an impending heart attack. However, when the three of us discussed what was happening, it was Elaine who had some additional helpful insights. She pointed out a pattern of changed behavior over the previous months—increased irritability, which was unusual for Robert, and diminished sexual activity. Elaine has had less trouble accepting the diagnosis of panic disorder than Robert. In fact, she welcomed it because it offered both an explanation and an expectation of recovery.

Robert would rather have retreated into the unending series of tests, x-rays, scans, and consultations that so often are prescribed for people with the symptoms of anxiety disease. Elaine helped him understand that it was okay for him to have an anxiety disorder, that it was a respectable disease, that she still idolized him as a man just as she always had. She encouraged him to get whatever help he needed. Without her insistence Robert would probably have discontinued the treatment as soon as he began to feel better.

Robert had a safe place where he felt comfortable, but where he also received some gentle, but firm, direction. It was a place where his natural tendency toward denial was not acceptable.

When Paul decided to accept early retirement it was a decision he and Edna made together. Then, when he developed anxiety symptoms, Edna provided the loving support he needed, as well as helpful insights. Paul's supportive home life allowed him to get through some difficult decisions and helped him grapple effectively with his health problems.

Gertrude was a neighbor of mine who may have died because of a home that gave her comfort but not encouragement; tolerance but not assistance. She had a lifelong fear of dentists. Gertrude was in her sixties when I first met her and had not had any dental work in her adult life. I only saw her one time as a patient when her own doctor was away. In the course of a brief examination I could not help but notice that she had only a few remaining badly decayed teeth in the front. The rest were still present, but only in the form of rotten, barely visible stumps.

I made what I thought was a tactful suggestion that perhaps a dentist—and she snapped a firm "no." Her husband told me later that she had always been afraid of dentists, and they had not discussed that subject in more than thirty years.

A few years later Gertrude developed throat cancer and died. The causes of throat cancer are largely unknown, but I do wonder if a half century of purulent infected drainage from rotting teeth may not have been the cause for Gertrude.

Gertrude had a place where she was appreciated, but not a home in the sense of nurturing, where she was encouraged to find ways to cope with problems constructively. Her family could have helped her find treatment for her phobia or an understanding dentist who would provide adequate medication and anesthesia to help her through the terror. Instead, there seemed to be a conspiracy of avoidance. A phobia that is permitted to constrict a person's life can be a dangerous disorder.

Henrietta felt comfortable at home, or at least, much more comfortable than when she tried to go out. Her mother accepted Henrietta's disability and never suggested going for help. Her doctor, my predecessor, told me he had once urged her to see a psychiatrist. He said she was astounded that he could suggest such a thing, "There's nothing wrong with my mind. I don't just imagine this moving feeling, it's real." Henrietta was amazed that with all of his years of experience, he didn't know better. She would not discuss it, and the topic was never again broached by either of them.

Henrietta's home was a place to hide. It was not a place where she was encouraged to get help. With no encouragement to grow, it was only a place to shrivel.

Everyone with an anxiety disorder needs a real home; we all do. But we need more than love, support, and acceptance. We also need nurturance and encouragement to grow. If you want to help a loved one with an anxiety disease, the best thing you can do is create, or be, that kind of home.

CARING FOR YOURSELF

Sara became a healing answer to Harry. But what about you and all the other would-be Saras of the world? You have been advised to learn about anxiety disease and encourage your friend to seek professional help to be certain of the correct diagnosis. This might require large doses of patience and persistence.

You've also been encouraged to be natural. This isn't easy, if your old inner tapes keep telling you to ignore symptoms that don't make sense or sound like childish fears.

You have been urged to be empathetic, to learn to be an active listener. This requires concentration, effort and, perhaps, learning new ways of relating to your spouse or friend.

All of these efforts may be emotionally draining. This is especially true if the person you are trying to help is the one you usually turn to for support and the one who has always made a home for you. Don't allow yourself to become a casualty. You can't help someone else up if you are down. Reach out for the support you need.

Your family doctor or a professional counselor can provide that support, as well as the information, advice, and encouragement both of you will need.

If you ask, your doctor may also know someone else with a similar problem who would be willing to share experiences with you. Or you may know other people in similar circumstances yourself. Talking with these people can be helpful, but only if you can do so without compromising your loved one's privacy.

Remember that trust and openness are part of the healing process. Let your loved one know you are concerned, how you feel, and what you are doing to help both of you. Honesty is not just the best policy, it is the only acceptable policy. An open and honest relationship will also help you stay healthy.

It should be a comfort to you to know that with treatment, your oved one's worst troubles should be shortlived. The knowledge that treatment works is another answer that heals.

SUMMARY

If your friend or loved one has anxiety disease you can take steps to create a supportive environment.

Be certain of the diagnosis. Anxiety disease can cause a variety of symptoms, but many other diseases can cause the same symptoms. Assist your friend in getting professional help to be sure.

You can help by:

- Being physically and emotionally available.
- Being as honest as you can without being controlling or judgmental.
- Offering help in any way needed.
- Being a source of security, understanding, and nurturing—a "home, sweet home."

Look after yourself; reach out for the support you need as well.

Hee is a better Physician that keepes diseases
off us, than he that cures them being on us.
Prevention is so much better than healing,
because it saves the labour of being sick.
                    Thomas Adams, 1612–1653 (Writer)

Chapter 15

Keeping the Snorklewackers
in the Closet

Humpty Dumpty sat on a wall,
Humpty Dumpty had a great fall . . .

Prevention is always better than treatment. Considering his delicate condition, Mr. Dumpty probably shouldn't have been sitting on a wall. Or maybe he should have used a seat belt or a helmet. Why did he fall? A slippery wall, the wind? Perhaps he had some internal problem that needed attention—a touch of salmonellosis or hypercholesterolemia?

Fortunately, if you have anxiety disease and become scrambled you can get yourself together again—and without all the king's horses and all the king's men.

As Mr. Dumpty would probably admit upon reflection, if he were able to reflect, preventing the problem is better than weathering it. We know the causes of anxiety disease are genetic, biological, and psychosocial. We don't know how to change our genetic heritage, and so far we still don't know what causes our anxiety chemistries to go out of kilter. Thanks to scientific advances in antianxiety medication, we have new insight into the causes of these diseases. With the hundreds of studies currently taking place, it seems likely that the basic biological

263

mechanisms behind anxiety diseases will soon be discovered. When that happens it should be possible to develop new ways of preventing anxiety disease from overwhelming us.

Meanwhile, we do know a great deal about the psychosocial causes of anxiety disease We know that we have the potential to learn to control many of them; to that extent, prevention is within our grasp.

Prevention can be either primary or secondary. For primary prevention you wear seat belts, get your immunizations, use smoke alarms, and if you are an egg, you don't sit on walls. In other words, primary prevention means doing or avoiding whatever is necessary to keep something bad from happening to you in the first place.

If something bad does happen, like cancer, diabetes, or gout, secondary prevention may help you find the cancer early enough to eradicate it or keep your diabetes from getting worse. It might prevent complications and keep you from having another attack of gout.

Mammography doesn't prevent breast cancer, but it can be a highly successful secondary preventive. With early detection, treatment may remove the disease. If you get diabetes, careful attention to diet and medication can help prevent heart damage or blindness.

If you have gout, preventing a recurrence might be as simple as following a diet or taking medication. Often the answer is education; we learn how to keep the same thing from happening again. If you are injured in a fire because you had no smoke detectors, you will make sure never to be without functioning smoke detectors again.

Unfortunately, you do not always have a second chance to un- scramble your life; if you are Humpty Dumpty, the best you can do is serve as someone's omelet.

Prevention of full-blown anxiety disease, both primary and sec- ondary, depends on some understanding of the causes of the disorder. What starts it, what makes it worse, and what causes complications or triggers recurrences? These factors can be internal or external. Possible internal factors for Mr. Dumpty might have included his naturally delicate condition, feeling ill and queasy, fear of heights, or simply the rotundity of his gluteus maximus. External factors could be a slippery wall, a windy day, or a purposeful shove by a bad egg.

In anxiety disorders there are also both internal and external causative factors. Each factor under our control is an opportunity to prevent anxiety disease.

The internal factors that caused Ruth's panic attacks were chemical or biological. Medication controlled those factors. First it relieved the anticipatory anxiety—that fear of another attack. Then it blocked the attacks completely.

In Hilda's case, the factors were both external and internal. The external factor was the milieu Max created; the internal factor was how she handled the situation. Her rehabilitation affected both factors. Max finally understood what was happening, which resulted in some change in his behavior (but probably not his basic attitude). Hilda's therapy helped her to understand their relationship better and demand a role in which she could be comfortable.

Primary prevention for Henrietta's anxiety disease might have been a shot-gun wedding (external) or some effective counseling when the disaster occurred. Secondary prevention could have been a nurturing home (external) and effective counseling and/or medication.

Many opportunities are available to prevent the exacerbation of anxiety disease because there are so many possible causative factors. Some prevention efforts can be effective both before and after the onset of the disease. Understanding the principles of primary and secondary prevention can help.

PRINCIPLES OF PRIMARY PREVENTION

Childhood Fears

Since one theory of the cause of phobias is that they may result from the persistence of normal childhood fears, we can help our children learn to resolve their fears when they are small. We do this through acknowledgment, support, openness, and sharing. For example, "I know you are afraid your closet is full of snorklewackers. Even though we turned on the light and looked, the scared feeling didn't go away. I'll stay with you until you feel better. With me it used to be tigers and horses. The tigers always hid under the table and the horses were under the bed. When I got a little older they all went away, but I'll tell you a secret—I still don't like horses very much."

This line of approach, in a quiet, affirming, supportive way, in small doses over a period of time, can help your child overcome the awful terrors that are often a part of childhood.

I had three great fears as a child, powerful enough to be vivid memories even now. My first fear was of dogs. I couldn't hide it because I ran inside whenever one was around. My father, a grocer, never made fun of me or tried to talk me out of it. He just chased any stray dog off with a banana stalk, always a handy weapon at that time. One day, while I was sitting in front of the store unwrapping oranges (they were all individually wrapped in red tissue), I suddenly became aware of something leaning over my shoulder, breathing in my face. It was a huge German shepherd. I was too scared to move, and the dog eventually wandered off. He could have separated my head from the rest of me as easily as I unwrapped oranges. I thought about that, realized that he hadn't, and my fear of dogs vanished.

That's how childhood fears are supposed to disappear. In a supportive environment we learn to separate real from imagined dangers.

My second big fear was of putting my head under water. I could hide this fear pretty well, except at camp. Every year, at considerable personal sacrifice (or so I thought, perhaps it was at considerable personal relief), my parents sent me to camp for two weeks. Since it meant so much to them, I always tried to be excited about going, and I could really have enjoyed it, except for my fear of water. I dreaded summer, because every year some counselor would try to get my head under water. One counselor was so disgusted with me she kept saying, "You make me sick." I felt guilty. She was a mean lady, but I didn't want to make her sick. If she died from her sickness it would be my fault. On the other hand, I wasn't willing to put my face in the water to sacrifice my life for hers.

That fear was badly handled and caused me unnecessary torment. I wasn't able to overcome it until high school. It would have been much better for me, and my counselor, if my fear had been openly accepted. If it had been, someone could have offered to help me with it or suggested some different water activities.

One afternoon when I was five, a cousin and I were playing outside when we heard a loud BANG. Since that was the loudest sound we had ever heard, we decided that the chocolate factory across the street had fallen down, but were too frightened to look. Then my dad came running out of the cellar carrying pieces of burning wood. Fire engines arrived and a great crowd gathered. My mother's first question was "What has my son done now?"

In reality, our furnace had exploded, setting off several small fires. No one was hurt and the fires were quickly extinguished. For many years after that I was terrified every time I was sent to the cellar on an errand. I always kept as much distance as possible between the furnace and me. When I had to pass it to go up the stairs, I always made a mad dash. When it blew up again, I wanted to be as far away from it as possible.

I never told anyone about those fears. It would have been unmanly and I was entering the first grade. As I grew those terrors gradually faded away. Had someone thought about how a little guy might react to an explosion in his home, and asked me about it, I would have had a lot to say. I might have admitted out loud how scared I was that the new furnace would blow up, too. I might also have had a much less traumatic period of adjustment.

When my wife and I had our own children we resolved to do better. One evening during a violent thunderstorm I was concerned that our smallest daughter might take on the same fear of storms her grandmother had lived with. So I commented, nonchalantly, that it sounded like God was moving the heavenly furniture around. To which our small daughter, sensing my concern, replied, "Yes, Daddy, and it must be hard to do with Jesus sitting on His right hand."

As parents we need to be aware of what our children do fear, and what they don't. They undoubtedly have several fears and they may be equally irrational but entirely different from our own. Our daughter had no fear of thunderstorms, although she suspected I had, but she did have other fears.

Honesty, openness, and time together may be all our children need to learn to grow through their fears. But if they seem to be having difficulty, professional help now might spare them an anxiety disease later.

Stress Management

Human existence is full of stress. It always has been, at least mythologically, since Pandora peeked into the box and Eve nibbled the apple. We are fond of saying that stress is the result of our modern, fast-paced civilization. There is no evidence that this is true. In fact, the stress levels that contribute to anxiety disease are just as intense in remote African villages. If we did not have the stress of competition, budgets, relationships, nuclear threats, environmental deterioration, and wild animals, we would probably suffer from the stress of boredom.

Eliminating all stress is neither a practical nor a desirable goal. Stress is not the main cause of our difficulties. In itself it is neither good nor bad, noxious nor nurturing. The problem is our response to stress.

It is our reaction that either does the mischief or stimulates us to be more effective in whatever we are trying to do.

We may use the stress of driving in Labor Day traffic to be alert, careful drivers. The anxiousness before the big game or competition may similarly spur us to do our best. The anxiousness of making a speech may help us hone our performance skills. As alertness, or anxiousness, increases, so does efficiency—up to a maximum point. And that is the catch. After the top of the curve, more anxiousness pushes us over the edge, down the other side. We then become too nervous to drive or too shaky to hold the notes for the speech. We drop the easy pass.

What each of us needs to learn is the ability to perceive when we are nearing the peak of our performance curve. We need to learn when to get help to manage our anxiousness, before we go over the edge.

We can also develop simple techniques to extend that performance curve. Driver training experience, physical conditioning, preparation, and rehearsal can all help decrease anxiousness and extend the performance curve.

Good anxiety can stimulate us to boost and enrich our efforts.

Avoidance, not denial, is the very best way to deal with many stresses. We may decide not to live on the edge of an active volcano, drive on Labor Day weekend, or join every protest. Not every confrontation requires a shootout. One of the basic lessons of martial arts is that, no matter how skillful and powerful you are, it is always better to walk away from a fight than attack. Linus van Pelt, Charlie Brown's philosopher friend, goes even further, "No problem is too big to run away from." Some stressful situations can be foreseen and avoided; some can be recognized and simply ignored; some can be evaded.

Some stresses, nevertheless, must be confronted. We must face them head-on, solve the problem, put out the fire, or chastise the troublemaker. However, most stresses, even those within our power to control, are more complicated than that. Even if they require a long-term solution, developing a plan and putting it into action can do wonders to relieve the anxiety that stress engenders.

Bert had an anxiety disorder related to his threatened job loss, which resulted in a problem of sexual dysfunction. When he and Polly worked out a plan to handle the possible unemployment, the symptoms of his anxiety disease disappeared.

Impending stress may become more manageable, and less anxiety producing, after effecting a plan to address whatever problems can be identified as causing the stress. Even before the plan is fully implemented, the stress will diminish.

However, if the anxiousness has already become an anxiety disease, decision making itself becomes a problem, which in turn exacerbates the stress. If we cannot run away, combat, or solve the object of stress, then we must cope with it. Throughout life, each of us learns different coping strategies. Some of them work and many of them don't. Since there seems to be an unlimited supply of stresses, we always need to be on the lookout for different and better ways of managing our responses.

One of my friends is an executive in a large corporation. He is often subject to stress, usually related to his boss, the CEO. This has been especially true during the company's peak season in the summer time. He eventually learned that a walk in the local countryside between the tall rows of corn was a good way for him to cope. It gave him isolation, a breath of fresh air, and solace. But one afternoon in the middle of the field, he looked up, startled to find himself face to face with his boss, who was doing the very same thing—and probably in response to the same situation.

One of my patients found that sweeping works best for her. It exercises the large muscles, and provides distraction and a sense of achievement. She has a lively household, but her floors, porch, sidewalks, and street are always immaculate.

Another woman baked cakes. Her family was constantly embroiled in dramatic events—violence, health crises, and interactions with the law. So she baked many cakes, usually coconut layer cake with coconut icing. My staff loved her. I am not sure whether it was the activity of baking that helped her most, or the pleasure of giving, but either way it worked for her.

Recently I gave a talk about stress to a group of elderly people in a retirement center. They listened politely, but impassively. I wasn't sure I really had their attention until I asked the question, "How do you handle the anxiousness that comes from stress?" That struck a chord and they all began talking about what worked for them. The ideas covered a broad spectrum including reading, fishing, praying, walking, visiting a friend who needed a friend, going for a drive, and listening to music. Their responses demonstrated how pervasive anxiousness as a response to stress is, and how each of us has developed personal mechanisms for coping.

There are many other successful coping techniques. Exercise is one of the very best. Golf, for example, uses most of the body's major muscle groups. It has the added advantage of allowing you to release anger and frustration by whacking a little ball, perhaps with the illusion that the boss's face is on it. Many other sports can do the same. The one major caution I have, other than staying within the limits of your physical fitness, is the reminder that if you have panic disorder, exercise can bring on an attack.

Meditation is another successful way of relieving the anxiousness of unresolved stress. Although previously described as a form of therapy for anxiety disease, it is probably most effective in preventing stress from leading to overwhelming anxiousness or triggering an anxiety disease. To be effective as a prophylactic, meditation should be practiced on a regular basis. One reason for this is that the benefits of meditation are cumulative; meditating regularly can help you develop resistance to the effects of stress. The other reason is that if you don't meditate regularly, at times of special stress it will not be as easy to slide into the process. You may be too anxious to focus on the process of meditating.

All of these are constructive ways people cope with the stresses of life. There are just as many destructive ways. Some are merely ineffective, some depend on trampling others, and some are self-destructive.

Excesses of alcohol, tobacco, or other drugs are obvious attempts to cope with stress. Some people eat voraciously whenever under stress, often compounding the problem with gastrointestinal discomfort or weight gain.

Some people, either consciously or unconsciously, take out their frustrations and anxieties resulting from stress on anyone who will tolerate it or can't fight back. This is the pecking-order-of-chickens or kick-the-dog syndrome.

Other poorly adaptive coping mechanisms are more subtle. Denial is a frequent, usually temporary, escape from stress. Pretend the problem doesn't exist and maybe it will go away. Workaholism is another. "I solved the last crisis by working harder. Now I just have to work harder. Twelve hours a day is a lot, but maybe I can work even faster and stay a little longer." This device has some seductive benefits. You are too distracted to think about your basic problem and huge amounts of work will be accomplished. The members of your family (if they are still around) should be pleased to have the extra money, and your boss is delighted (and already planning ways to increase your productivity another five percent next year).

Clearly there are many ways of dealing with stress, but we still have much to learn. While stress is one of the major problems of living, perhaps of survival, it seems tragic to me that it is rarely addressed in our educational system. We teach driver's education courses to encourage basic survival techniques. We emphasize sports in our schools as a means of competing with each other, and as a way of improving our status at the expense of others. Never are sports applauded for the sheer joy of exercise, or encouraged as a means of self-expression, or promoted as a way of coping with stress. Even in music and art, our emphasis tends to be on competition and performance, not appreciation or self-expression. We teach simple health rules like don't smoke, don't drink, don't do drugs, don't have premarital sex, use a condom if you do, eat the basic four food groups, sleep eight hours, etc. But we fail to teach the basic lessons of living a healthy life, such as communication skills, forging healthy relationships, and coping with the stress of being human.

Anxiety diseases are caused by biological or psychosocial factors, or both. Stress is a psychosocial factor: how we handle it can help us protect ourselves from one of the causes of anxiety disease.

There is another way you can partially protect yourself against anxiety disease. Following Mom's advice may be good for your health, although it may sound like the school hygiene course you slept through. I am, however, certain that attention to these dull details will contribute to your overall sense of well being.

Caffeine, alcohol, tobacco, and other drugs all affect the anxiety response. Caffeine tends to increase anxiety symptoms. So does tobacco, but less so in a person who is addicted enough to have developed a tolerance. Alcohol relieves anxiety symptoms initially, but then becomes a depressant for many people. Other drugs such as marijuana and cocaine each carry their own set of ills. Generally, caffeine and alcohol in moderation are safe.

A balanced diet can do wonders. This includes what you eat and when you eat it. Choose a variety of foods from within the food groups; eating many different things will please your body and your palate. Eating frequent, small meals is better for you than only one big meal. Your diet should be high in complex carbohydrates (eat your vegetables!) and low in fat. It should have enough fiber so that your stools float.

Requirements for water vary enormously. No one can tell you

exactly how much you need. A good guideline, however, is to drink enough fluids to keep your urine pale in color.

Sleep is also essential but variable among groups of people. Young people need more sleep than older people. You need enough sleep to feel rested in the morning.

Exercise is extremely important, but how much of what kind do you need? As a general guideline, do enough stretching exercises so that you feel limber in the morning. Do enough muscle building exercises to be as strong as you want to be. Do enough aerobic exercise so that you can climb a flight of stairs without huffing. And don't forget to do some of your exercise outside. Mom was right. You need fresh air and sunshine as part of a balanced life.

There is one more thing that Mom probably practiced, but may not have recognized as essential to good health—affection. The importance of affection to good health, even to survival, was discovered many years ago in studies investigating why some orphaned infants in an institution in France did poorly while others in the same institution did well. In one ward the babies were given all of the physical essentials, but were not handled any more than necessary to get the work accomplished. In another ward the same basic care was provided, but the nurses were in the habit of holding, snuggling, and interacting with each of their little charges. In the first ward many of the infants failed to thrive and some died, but all did well in the second ward. Researchers documented a vivid and important lesson for us all.

More recent studies in adult men showed that the absence of loving support can be an important risk factor for heart disease.

Our health to some extent depends on developing loving relationships, and building a home as a refuge.

PRINCIPLES OF SECONDARY PREVENTION

Secondary prevention means keeping the illness you have from getting worse. Secondary prevention keeps an acute problem, like adjustment disorder, from becoming a chronic problem, like generalized anxiety disorder. It also means preventing complications like having panic disorder lead to agoraphobia or an anxiety disorder lead to depression. When you have recovered from anxiety disorder, secondary prevention means preventing a recurrence or, if it should start, nipping it in its nasty bud.

Generalized anxiety disorder tends to be chronic, with flare-ups of symptoms from time to time. Knowing what to do at the very start can save you much grief. Agatha, who struggled with her anxiety disorder for more than thirty years, finally learned to recognize the early symptoms. Now she calls me as soon as anything begins to go wrong.

Panic disorder also has a propensity for recurrence. The attacks are easier to recognize, but it is crucial to deal with them promptly. Robert, whose panic attacks began with chest pain, finally accepted the diagnosis of panic disorder. He did not want to take any kind of medication, but he finally agreed to do so, on an ongoing basis, for several months. Once he was symptom free, we tried tapering off the drug several times, but each time he began to have symptoms—not major panic attacks but limited symptom attacks. However, he recognized what was happening and by increasing the dose, again became symptom-free. He now continues to be symptom-free on a small maintenance dose.

There are four general principles of secondary prevention, although the first two are exactly the same as in primary prevention.

The first is, find a home, a refuge. Hilda finally was able to do this after her rehabilitation. While her home might not be ideal, she is comfortable in it. She feels supported, encouraged, and reasonably understood by Max. Bert and Polly, who came face to face with their deteriorating home because of sexual dysfunction, were able to repair the damage together. Frank and Francine's relationship never recovered from "that damn trip to Washington." Frank continues to suffer the consequences, and Francine continues to skim through life as if no problems existed.

The second is, do what Mom said. This may have been an important part of David's recovery. David joined a commune for nearly two years, where he found the home, affection, and nurturance he needed. The health rules of the commune were fairly rigid, at least concerning diet, drugs, and exercise. This may have been an integral part of David's recovery, since he needed guidance in all three areas. Professional help, however, would almost certainly have made David's recovery more rapid and more sure.

The third principle concerns treatment as prevention. One goal of treatment is for you to feel better and to be rid of all of your miserable symptoms. A second goal is to keep the symptoms away.

If you are like many of us, when your symptoms first appeared, you tried to pretend that they weren't significant, and would go away by themselves. Often the symptoms do disappear for awhile, thereby "proving" you were right. When they return you try to deny their existence again, since it worked the last time. Eventually with anxiety disorders, the symptoms cannot be ignored; you know you must do something to get relief. Ernie DeWitt, the beloved high school coach, had trouble believing there was anything wrong, and even more trouble learning that he could not overcome it through strength of will or faith.

Treatment works. When it helps quickly, as it often does with medication, there is a great temptation to stop taking the drugs. Common responses are: "I'm okay now and probably didn't even need the drug." "I feel like my old self; I'll just keep thinking more positive and get on with my life." "My prayers were answered. I can forget all about that psychology stuff and drugs."

This kind of logic may seem absurd or irrational, but *only* to those who have never experienced an anxiety disorder. Remember that the symptoms of anxiety disease are often bizarre, not the customary symptoms of flu, ulcers, or arthritis.

When the symptoms seem peculiar, the stricken person often finds it is much easier and more acceptable to pretend that they didn't really happen at all. This attitude of denial is aided and abetted by the guilt, that inner certainty that anyone should be able to handle this alone. When the symptoms disappear, people convince themselves that they were right. There is danger in this response.

If your symptoms disappear, it does not mean that the underlying illness is gone. Something needs to be fixed or you surely will have more suffering. The nature of anxiety disease is such that the next batch of symptoms could be different, and perhaps even more disturbing than the first.

Psychosocial problems may be the cause, or a contributing cause, of your anxiety disorder. Even with excellent counseling, sorting these out and addressing them is rarely a quick process. Treatment takes time to work. If you are taking medication, that, too, takes time to work.

In some conditions, adjustment disorder or performance anxiety, for example, you may be advised to take medications only when you need them. With most anxiety disorders, however, medications are prescribed for regular use. You may feel that the dose is wrong for you. Perhaps there are too many side effects or the dose is too small to achieve the desired effect. If so, call your doctor immediately and discuss it. Everyone is different and we all respond differently to drugs. Only you can know what you feel. If you are taking medications regularly, especially the short-acting BZDs like Xanax or Ativan, there is also the danger of an immediate flare-up of symptoms if you stop abruptly. These drugs should always be tapered off gradually.

The medications available for anxiety disease, and for depression, are potent. They can do wonderful things for you, but they can also cause you more trouble if not taken properly. Both counseling, to help you unwind life's tangles, and drugs, used wisely, can help you recover without complications and help you stay well.

The final principle is to know yourself and your treatment program. One of the major challenges of life is learning to know yourself. Sometimes this is exhilarating, sometimes upsetting, but it is always full of surprises. The first encounter with anxiety disorder is a new experience. To get better and stay better, you need to consider several points.

You will need to have a maintenance plan. If you are taking medication for your anxiety disorder, you need to know under what circumstances you should change the dose, either up or down, what long-term side effects are possible, and when and how to stop. For many people with anxiety disorders drugs are used from several weeks to several months and then discontinued. Both generalized anxiety disorder and panic disorder, however, have a tendency to recur. For these, the treatment that works best can be used whenever there is a flare-up. In a few people, recurrences of symptoms are so frequent that it is wisest to continue on a small maintenance dose of medication indefinitely.

With counseling you also need a long-term plan. The purpose of counseling is to help you understand the complexities of your psychosocial self, and to deal with your problems. How long you should continue counseling and how deep you should probe will depend on the type and seriousness of the difficulties you find, and how much you feel the need for outside help to handle them.

Hilda went far enough in therapy to manage her addictive problem and work out an acceptable relationship with Max. She chose not to try to change herself so drastically that she would be entirely independent of him.

Agatha has had many flare-ups of symptoms over a period of thirty years. The best plan she and I were able to work out is a low-maintenance dose of drugs and regularly scheduled visits every six weeks. These visits permit me to check on symptoms, monitor her medication, and offer some basic counseling. When she has any symptoms between visits, she reports them by telephone and an interim visit is arranged if needed; more often, she simply needs reassurance.

Mr. Elsworth Jones, the pompous man with both anxiety disease and heart disease, could have benefited by following a maintenance plan, for both problems. Mr. Jones would come to the office only rarely and for nonurgent visits. When confronted with this he always said it was because he already owed me so much money, which was true. I was never able to convince him that prevention would have been cheaper than treatment.

Edith is my friend from out of town who had seen sixteen doctors in almost as many specialties in a two-year period. Once the correct diagnosis was established, she needed a maintenance plan more than anything else. We worked out a plan for weekly visits at first, then monthly visits for the combined purpose of counseling and monitoring her medications. I also extracted from her, with some difficulty, the solemn promise that no matter what new symptoms may develop, she will call me first before dashing off for another series of work-ups. This has worked well for several years.

If you have a long-term anxiety disease, stay in close touch with some professional who can help you. If you are planning to move, or your physician or counselor plans to move, be sure to establish a new relationship beforehand. As Charles Henry Webb asked in the last century, is it not wiser, "To be sure that they are on with the new love before being off with the old?" This is good advice for those with any serious illness that may flare up, but especially those suffering from anxiety diseases. The stress of the move itself, or the loss of an esteemed professional and friend, could precipitate more symptoms. Having a maintenance plan can be so effective in staving off another attack; it seems foolish, but very human, not to have one.

Part of knowing yourself is knowing your limits. We all have limits. We have physical limits, like knowing when to stop playing football with the neighborhood kids. We have intellectual limits, like trying to understand the legal fine print on the maintenance plan for the new computer. And we have emotional limits. How much can I handle before my increasing anxiety shoves me over the edge of the curve?

Learning our limits is a difficult lesson for all of us. It ought to become easier as we get older, but it does not seem to. Bobby Riggs was sure he could beat any woman tennis player. Frank thought he could force himself into the elevator at the Washington Monument, but he could not—even in the face of public derision.

The other part of knowing your limits is anticipating those limits. Anticipating limits gives you options.

You may be able to avoid the stressor: Don't go to Washington; don't perform if you are not ready; don't sit on a wall if you are an egg. To avoid what you know you cannot tolerate is not "wimping out"; it is using your intellect. Don't let "them," or anyone, coerce you into trying to do what you know you cannot do. Only you can know your limits.

A second option is to desensitize yourself. If the stress can be meted out in small doses, you might get used to it. With professional support, Frank managed to get to the third floor of the department store before Francine discouraged him from continuing therapy.

If you anticipate your limits, you also have the option of arming yourself against an attack through preparation. The better the preparation, the less the anxiety. This is most obviously true with performance anxiety. If I do not prepare thoroughly for a public presentation, I will be uncomfortably anxious, and with good reason, because I probably will not do well.

Preparation for other kinds of stress can also be helpful. If you have an anxiety disease and know a crisis is coming that will tax the limits of your tolerance, you can gather all of your coping tools. Review what you have learned in counseling in terms of your strengths and specific skills. You might even want to begin your anxiolytic medication before dealing with the crisis. You might also want to discuss the impending situation with your doctor or counselor.

Preparation was a great support to Joan, my patient who wanted to go with her husband on fishing trips, but could not force herself to go and could not even make a decision about what to wear. When she improved she again considered the possibility of an overnight trip. We worked out a plan to increase her medication forty-eight hours before each venture. It worked like a charm and after three or four trips she no longer needed to take the extra medication. She still carries it along, though, because "It's a comfort just to know it's there."

YOUR FUTURE

Remember that the answers that heal, all of them, apply directly to you.

You are not alone. Thirteen million other adult Americans have also had an anxiety disorder within the past six months. Anxiety disorders are not peculiarly American. They affect all people alive today and all who have gone before us. Until we find a truly reliable "immunization" they will continue to be with us. Two out of every twenty people you know probably have an anxiety disorder. Who are they? As with most other illnesses, once you acknowledge you have it, you will hear about it from dozens of others. But beware of well-meaning people who need to tell you horror stories. "Aunt Mamie had exactly the same thing and they locked her up for thirty years."

Be assured that you are not alone (although, with too many Aunt Mamie stories, you might rather be).

The second answer that heals is that *it is not your fault*. You did not cause this disease to befall you, either because of something you did or something you failed to do. You do need to recognize, however, that other people, who have no personal experience with anxiety disorders, may not know that. You may want to share your new knowledge with them.

The other answer that heals is that *treatment works*. With medication or counseling, usually both, you *can* recover. Treatment is safe and the side effects are usually innocuous and manageable. If cost is an over-riding concern, ask your doctor to choose a medication available in generic form. If counseling is too costly, check with your local mental health clinic.

Remember that you are not Humpty Dumpty. He sat on a wall alone. That was a poor decision in his fragile condition, and his ensuing disorder, the fall, was unfixable. But you are a person. And you are not alone. You are in great company; you didn't cause your trouble—and you can get well and stay well.

SUMMARY

Primary prevention is doing or avoiding whatever is necessary to keep something bad from happening to you.

Since one theory holds that some phobias are the result of persistent childhood fears, we can help our children resolve those fears.

Stress management is essential. We can respond to stress in several ways:

We can use it to improve performance up to a point.

Many stresses can be avoided.

Some stresses can be confronted.

We can cope with stress in constructive ways including exercise and meditation.

Following the basic "Mom knows best" principles will have good effects on your health.

If something bad does happen, *secondary prevention* may help you to recognize the problem early enough to eradicate it, keep it from getting worse, or keep it from happening again.

- Find a home, a refuge.
- Do what Mom said.
- Treatment is a form of prevention.
- Know yourself, your limits, and your treatment program.

These are the answers that heal:

- You are not alone.
- It's not your fault that you have anxiety disease.
- Treatment works—you can get well and stay well.

Further Reading

Benson, Herbert, *The Relaxation Response* (New York: William Morrow & Co., Inc., 1975).
Fried, Barbara, *Who's Afraid? The Phobic's Handbook*, rev. ed. (New York: Gardner Press, 1985).
Greist, John H., James W. Jefferson, and Isaac M. Marks, *Anxiety and Its Treatment* (Washington, D.C.: American Psychiatric Press, Inc., 1986).
Henley Arthur, *Phobias: The Crippling Fears* (New York: Lyle Stuart, 1987).
LeShan, Lawrence, *How To Meditate* (Boston: Little, Brown & Co., 1974).
Nathan, Ronald G., Thomas E. Staats, and Paul J. Rosch, *The Doctors' Guide to Instant Stress Relief* (New York: G. P. Putnam & Sons, 1987).
Sheehan, David V., *The Anxiety Disease* (New York: The Scribner Book Companies, 1983).
Weekes, Claire, *Hope and Help for Your Nerves* (New York: Hawthorne Books, Inc., 1969).

Notes

1. J. B. Cobb, How to Cope with Anxiety, *Postgraduate Medical Journal*, 58:623–629 (1982).
2. Berke Breathed, *Penguin Dreams and Stranger Things* (Boston, Toronto: Little, Brown and Company, 1985), p. 89.
3. Thomas H. Holmes and Richard H. Rahe, The Social Readjustment Rating Scale, *Journal of Psychosomatic Research*, 11:216 (1967).
4. David V. Sheehan, *The Anxiety Disease* (New York: The Scribner Book Companies Inc., 1983), pp. 33–34. (Reprinted with permission of Charles Scribner's Sons, an imprint of Macmillan Publishing Company from *The Anxiety Disease* by David V. Sheehan, M.D. Copyright 1983 by David V. Sheehan.)
5. J. A. Ewing, Detecting Alcoholism, the CAGE Questionnaire, *Journal of the American Medical Association*, 252:1905–1907 (1984).
6. L. Covi and R. S. Lipman, Primary Depression or Primary Anxiety? A Possible Psychometric Approach to a Diagnostic Dilemma, *Clinical Neuropsychopharmacology*, 7:924–925 (1984).
7. R. S. Lipman, Differentiating Anxiety and Depression in Anxiety Disorders: Use of Rating Scales, *Psychopharmacology Bulletin*, 18(4):69–77 (1982).
8. Claire Weekes, *Hope and Help for Your Nerves* (New York: Hawthorne Books, Inc., 1969).

Index

www.ingramcontent.com/pod-product-compliance
Ingram Content Group UK Ltd.
Pitfield, Milton Keynes, MK11 3LW, UK
UKHW022304280225
455674UK00001B/157